Lesbian Erotica

Short BDSM LGBT Romance Why Choose A
Reverse Harem

Terrence Meza

Are you turning up the heat by one or two degrees? You are either also a lesbian, bisexual, or really inquisitive. I've never seen you dressed the way you do before. And even if you toned it down that day, your confidence persisted. I have never seen you seem so confident. Everyone was taking a second look after you. I'll confess that seeing everyone swoon over you made me feel a little envious, but how could I blame them?

You certainly have a strong work ethic. At least you have limited your inspection to ladies exclusively now. You caught me gazing at you again, but there was no way I stood out more than the rest since I had the same expression and thoughts going through my brain as everyone else had.

I'm delighted you made the decision to keep doing whatever it is. Though being under your control makes me feel a bit uneasy, I know you make each day better for me. I'm not sure whether this is the day you decide one way or the other, but I'm going to take advantage of it while I can.

Section Five

Okay, you have become purely wicked. I am aware that you are making an effort to tease me, and it is effective. Although you can't see me, you are making me flinch. Are you loving this power trip you're having? Now that you know you have me in your grasp, you don't even try to seek for me anymore. God, I need to rein in my thoughts. You probably got the idea as I was thinking about my fingers and your fingertips.

After seeing you, it's tough for me to focus on anything. I believe that we are playing a game with each other, thus I feel as if I have gained some insight into you. You like rivalry. You assume that before you do, I will give in to my wants. You anticipate that I will approach you if I give in to my weakness. So go sexy, game on! I'm also a natural competitor. Give it your best and go for it. Bring your best effort, but heed my warning: you are going down. I want to descend, hold on a second. It's possible that the sexual tension is getting to me, but whomever can hold off the longest will be rewarded for every agonizing temptation that pushes the boundaries of my resolve.

Paragraph 2

After six months, the ladies had developed incredible friendships. They had been exploring pubs, theaters, and other entertaining locations. When not at work, they spent a lot of time together and had developed a few inside jokes. They also made jokes about slapping one other's bums and made comments about each other's body. When they gathered, they were a little riot.

Kim was preparing for a new day. She got out of bed, performed some morning yoga, cleaned her teeth, and grabbed a smoothie that had already been prepared before leaving for work. As soon as she entered, she realized it would be another exhausting day. She said, "I'm going to need another girls' night."

A busload of children were in the emergency room sobbing, screaming, and running about because a bus and a large Ford had crashed somewhere in the town. She took a quick glance around before going to the locker room to change and get ready for work. It would have been lovely if she had sipped her smoothie. As she removed her clothes, she pulled an earring, which hurt. Of course, she also had to cope with the ridiculous spotting that had begun two days into her cycle. The day was going to be wonderful.

She headed straight for the work desk as she re-entered the emergency room. Staci quickly got her to work checking in children who hadn't yet been accepted. She quickly went to her first child and was herself. She turned to face the little child, who had a small cut along his jaw line and a hot itch on his cheek. To it, he was clutching a tissue.

Hello, I'm Kim, and it's lovely to meet you.

Although he was crying a little, the little youngster nevertheless managed to say hello.

"What's your name, buddy?"

The little child started to announce his name before blurting out, "Mommy!" A lady ran over and started sobbing. Which sparked the children's agitation? She started to panic out as she held her kid, but Kim swiftly stopped her.

She said, "Hi, I'm Kim, is this your son?" She gave a nod. The youngster was weeping and holding her at the time. Kim completed the chart as soon as she obtained all the information she need on the child.

The mother said, "When can a doctor see my son?"

After pausing, Kim was going to inform the woman that it would take a while when she felt a strong touch on her shoulder. When she turned around, Alison was grinning and said, "Right now, actually."

Kim promptly introduced herself and grinned before returning to her workstation to properly admit the patient. The remainder of the morning continued in the same manner, with nurses frantically admitting patients and physicians quickly providing care.

Working almost side by side with Alison all day was pleasant, in Kim's opinion.

A few hours had gone by the time everyone had been admitted, the last patients had been treated, and more people were still arriving throughout the day. When there was finally a break, Kim rested her head on the edge of the desk to collect her breath. After taking off her latex gloves, Alison approached and handed them some paperwork. She then sighed while leaning on the desk.

Staci replied, completing one file before taking the next from the apparently endless stack of work. "Good work out there you two," she added.

Alison said, "Same to you, so, drinks tonight?"

Staci apologized, "No can do, I have to get home and see my little girl."

Kim exclaimed, "I'm in," and "Should we invite Jenn and Mike?"

Then turning around, Alison straightened her back. Already inquired, seems to be just the two of us tonight.

"That sounds good. When do you leave?"

Alison glanced at the time and said, "About two hours."

She said, taking a pen and paper, "Great, I'm done in an hour," and scrawled a name on the pad. Meet me here, and when you enter, I'll have a drink waiting for you.

I'll see you there, Alison said while grabbing the letter.

By all accounts, O'Brady's bar had a wonderful setting. It was a little too quiet and tranquil to draw in the neighborhood frat guys, yet a bit too loud and rapid for the more mature population. A fantastic pocket was left for the 25–35 audience. When Alison entered, Kim was tossing darts. She leaned towards the throw as the dart exited her palm. Her body was well complemented by her tight pants. As she rose from the toss, her long brown hair streamed back and forth. She saw Alison carefully scanning the area out of the corner of her eye.

The blonde lady responded, "Nice throw," while giving her buddy a cat-like look. She had just started to notice Kim in a manner that aroused her. Her grin, that bouncy, rhythmic voice. Not even to mention the way she moved. She has such young vigor and a definite spring in her stride.

She stepped up and pulled the dart out in the wooden paneling a few inches away from the board, saying, "Thanks, though the beer I've had didn't really help." They moved over to a little booth where Alison was holding a drink.

How was the date you had with Gregg, was that it? As she sipped her drink, Alison remarked.

Ah, that! Yeah, it didn't go so well," she chuckled as pictures of the terrible incident played.

After giving her companion a pat on the shoulder, Alison relaxed and let her arm fall over her shoulders. Kim related to her the tale of Gregg, who was a genuinely wonderful man, how their first date over coffee went well, and how Gregg also much enjoyed their pleasant second date. Everything was extremely great. She terminated it because it was going nowhere and she wanted fun, not polite.

Alison chugged her drink and set the glass down on a coaster. "Well, there's always more fish in the sea," she replied. Kim gave her a moment of attention before laughing.

What is that? She laughed inconsolably as she continued, "Some corny romance story.

If the shoe fits properly, she muttered. I'm going to fetch another, would you want one?

Alison approached the bar while keeping Kim's attention on her shoulder as Kim nodded. In her little too tight dress pants, Alison walked. With each stride, her slender legs and behind swayed. Her cropped jacket matched the length of her hips and highlighted her physique. Kim coveted her friend's full physique since she was so envious of it.

She went back to the booth and sat down after transferring Kim's drink. They raised their glasses in celebration of all those possible newcomers. Though I suppose there were times when fishing in a nearby pond was simpler. For a time, the ladies engaged in conversation and laughter before returning to the darts. When Kim became interested, they engaged in a few games.

Kim said, "Hey Alison," in an interested but somewhat terrified voice, "So, gynecology?"

That's what I do, she said.

"Is there a reason? It would have required real enthusiasm to have produced enough work to have a speciality, right?

Alison positioned her drink on an adjacent table and said, "So?"

"I just wanted to know if you..." Without really knowing where she was heading with this, Kim stumbled.

"Really?" Hearing this statement again made Alison a bit more than irritated. She had heard it throughout medical school and could quickly recognize it. When questioned, everyone spoke in the same tone. Every single. Time. Are you a lesbian? You want to know that, right?

Kim stuttered, caught but still interested, "Well, no, I mean...yeah." She requested with a bent head and apologized. She was inquisitive but didn't want to insult Alison. Kim had a natural interest in women and even adopted the typical collegiate curiosity.

Then, with a square shoulder and a hint of rage, Alison turned to face her. Up until that moment, Kim had been a nice friend, and Alison understood she needed to remain open-minded. "So, why do you ask, then?"

Since we've spent a lot of time together and I like you, Alison, I was simply wondering. Kim stopped, hesitant to reveal her but yet willing to take a risk.

Alison took a step back and saw her buddy shrink herself in front of her. Kim bit her lip as she glanced up at her. In the short time they had known one other— just six months—they had become incredibly close friendships. superior than anybody Alison has ever encountered. Why would she ask her to do such a thing? In front of herself, Alison acknowledged having

Are you proposing to me? In order to seem confident, Alison inquired while arched-eyed.

Kim's lips curled into a little grin at the corner. Then, she took a little more pride in Alison's comprehension and stood higher. She gave her pal a direct glance before bursting into her upbeat, jovial speech. "And what if I am?"

Alison was a bit taken aback by the petite brunette firecracker's direct manner of delivering it. As she gained confidence, she almost came across as cocky.

The sophisticated lady raised her glass and sipped from it while maintaining an intense eye contact with Kim. She gave the idea some thinking. The little woman, who was also her friend, had given her more pleasure during the previous six months than any other person she had interacted with. But isn't that what true friends are like?

She started off by saying, "Kim, I've, never," not wanting to tell her friend no but also not wanting to say no.

They both felt wonderful after a few beers and a fun night out, and Kim had an idea? "How about we try it instead of just saying no?" Although a bit taken aback by her own bravado, Kim maintained her composure.

After taking a drink of her beer, she said, "So, I know we have Wednesday off next week. Let's leave work together, get ready, and then go on a date. She slightly leaned to the right, allowing her hip to protrude so her leg could be seen. The boys always benefited from it. She muttered a little, "Worse comes to worth," She shook her head and waved her palm forth to emphasize the present excursion, saying, "It looks like two girls hanging out like we are right now."

Alison contemplated it. Her mind then wandered to a young lad. When Tom was young, she had a close friend who want to date. He was a decent child, but he struggled to let things go when they didn't work out. She never saw him again after they immediately stopped communicating to one another. However, things were different with Kim. Never before has she felt so connected to another person. Even so, they made light of one another and had fun.

Why not, after all, they were already virtually dating. The blonde beauty has been to clubs and pubs like this on a good number of occasions. They drank and played darts. What's the distinction? Kim, at least, kept her companion from dozing off throughout the movies they watched. Oh, let's ignore it.

Let's go on our date and see how it goes, then. However, I don't want our relationship to become uncomfortable or strained if it doesn't work out.

Kim excitedly nodded her head. It won't since a handful of my ex-boyfriends are still close with me; don't worry, we can resolve the issue.

Alison felt a surge of anxious energy. Kim said, "We can figure it out." Alison grinned at the idea. It had always been about you or me, never about us or us. Perhaps the vibe wasn't nervous but rather excited.

With a few more beers, they ended their ladies' night. They eventually located the jukebox and started playing their old favorites. That evening, they both discovered that Alison had surgeon-like precision in her dart-throwing. She more than handled on her own despite the alcohol's ineffectiveness. The remainder of the evening was spent laughing and giggling as a newfound enthusiasm fueled them both.

Rosetta was excited in the vehicle when they departed. She was experiencing a noticeable adrenaline surge. She had probably only seen bar fights after they broke out, dealing with them as a police officer. She nearly participated in this one.

"Holy sh*t, Bellamy, those two battled for me! It's really unbelievable. They have no idea who I am.

"They had the information they needed. that you are appealing. they desired you." Bellamy sped past a sluggish car. Only those who were drunk, high on drugs, or elderly drove so slowly. She cast a quick check in her rearview mirror at the driver. The third explanation must be true since she saw a cloud of white hair. Or even the third in addition to either one or both of the others. You just didn't know.

In Bellamy's automobile, Rosetta was the passenger and she was kind of jumping about with more enthusiasm than she could contain. "You threw the tall one into the air as if you were some kind of superheroine. Lady Wonder. You're my hero, haha.

Bellamy was happy to be driving instead of Rosetta. Rosetta was buzzed on adrenaline despite not having had a drop of alcohol. When they left The Spinning Wheel earlier on their way to The Stray, Bellamy had directed it—no pun intended—so that they took her vehicle. Why? Dorothe had ordered her to make a modest movement. It would give Bellamy an undertone of "I'm driving, I'm in control" to go along with Rosetta's already existing undertone of "I need to make you happy to get this job I now covet."

Bellamy had a wave of guilt. culpability from before the fact. guilt for planning ahead. the kind of shame intended to persuade someone to modify their behavior before it was too late. Bellamy, though, felt completely powerless to alter direction.

In the same way that Dorothe controlled her in the bedroom, other places, and even the stupid bathroom, Dorothe also controlled her thoughts.

Even the thought of disappointing Dorothe or defying her was awful. Since her fifth-grade love on Eric Sheehan, she hadn't experienced anything like.

Super Bell-a-meeeee! Rosetta crooned out loud in a mock-hushed announcer's voice during the short pause.

Rosetta, fuck you. Only surprise and leverage were used.

You're my superheroine, Rosetta beamed. You superheroines are all very humble. You kept me alive.

I did not protect you. They both desired you, and neither would have intended any harm. I prevented damage to the elder one. And I'm sure you could have dealt with anybody who had pursued you.

"Sure, that. However, nice work. What did you think, then? Is it going well? Did I come across as a nice lesbian? That's what I wanted to achieve.

"Good job, you. Over a female they believed to be heterosexual, they wouldn't fight.

19

Did you see how they were attempting to touch me, you know?

"I saw their success. You have great tolerance. You didn't flinch or behave in a manner that made you seem untrustworthy. Dorothe Gerbach frequents several lesbian clubs and mingles with their clientele. Bodyguards and even non-lesbian ladies are not permitted at some of those locations. Whatever happens, Dorothe will still leave, and it is our responsibility to follow. Even if she doesn't take all the necessary precautions to keep herself safe, she still needs to be safeguarded.

"Okay. I recognize."

"But that's not all. Remember, there are many ways we need to assist Dorothe. utter trash. Idiot crap. I hate to admit it, but we may sometimes aid in her seductions.

The question "What the fuck?"

Not in that way. We may have to divert him if she tries to seduce a straight woman who has a partner. Play the hit on him. or something like. Another possibility is a lesbian pair, in which case we would keep one occupied while Dorothe pursued the other.

"My God. To a lesbian seductress, like... henchmen or henchwomen?

"I believe you understand. Going above and above is a big part of our work.

But, you know, no genuine lesbian material, right?

You decide. A free world exists. No judgment here.

"Very amusing. But really, what if Ms. Gerbach flirts with me?

"Same response as before."

"Well, no, I'd say. All males are my favorites. All rules apply. Well, high school is not included.

It was fascinating. Maybe get her remembering and talking about their experience in high school? However, it can backfire if the recollection wasn't a nice one.

The question "Has Ms. Gerbach ever hit on you?"

Shit. Excellent query from Rosetta. Bellamy hated lying, but what else could she possibly say? Tell Rosetta that "Ms.

Gerbach" absolutely charmed her and that at this point, just a few days later, Bellamy was already "Ms. Gerbach's" lesbian sex slave and "Ms. Gerbach" was her mistress.

Better not tell her all that, I agree.

I don't want to discuss it, but I believe Ms. Gerbach finds me appealing.

Bellamy appreciated her response. Although it was mostly the truth, it was nonetheless the truth.

"I now know you're a trustworthy individual. If that's how she is, I knew she had to have had feelings for you. Who could blame a lesbian for falling for you, by the way? You are gorgeous. The lesbian in me would go for you. After all, you are my superheroine.

Saying "Jeez, stop." Bellamy really wished she would stop. Already, she felt much too bad. Bellamy felt like a lesser kind of creature the more Rosetta elevated her.

What now, future boss?

A good query. Bellamy was supposed to invite Rosetta on the dance floor as part of the original plan. Some close dancing and trial touching that wasn't too brazen were all allegedly part of the testing. Rosetta might get heated by it.

Perhaps Bellamy might still do it in her home. She was escorting Rosetta there. It had always been the intention to bring her there, just not this quickly or with Rosetta so sober.

In most cases, interacting with someone in a public place is limited. especially when it comes to Rosetta. Rosetta would already find it difficult to be seduced in alone, much less with other people there to make her feel even more exposed.

Bellamy was also required to employ a method or instrument in Dorothe's scheme that would not be popular with the general populace.

Handcuffs.

"Andrea, I can't believe how simple it is for women to leave the office because guys are too afraid to inquire as to what the issue is. Guys are extremely clueless, but I suppose that's part of their appeal. She had purposefully worn these really good denim pants that didn't cover anything when I was sitting on the bed watching her get ready. She even took off her spectacles and put in her contacts, giving her face a younger appearance, and I had the strangest impression that she was getting dressed to impress Tina.

"I won't advise you what to dress, but it seems like you've chosen to play up and emphasize all of your curves. Those pants cling so closely to your ass that even a tiny bend will offer the world a look they won't soon forget. Are you certain that you aren't simply doing this

24

to outdo me in terms of appearance, Andrea? You may be honest with me, but I wouldn't hold it against you. She was putting her trousers on before picking a beautiful pink t-shirt that displayed her toned breasts. We were both fortunate in that regard, and there were many occasions when we would glance at one another and realize that many females didn't have a chance in our presence.

"I'm just hoping to get off to a good start. I felt I had to somewhat compete after you complimented her beauty, ha ha. Sometimes it comes down to how you appear, so I simply want to highlight the fact that I'm coming with you. Since I didn't have a vehicle and didn't need one, I walked after her to get to hers. Almost everything was fair game for this girl, even meals that would make most people gag.

My chest began to feel hot, and I had to readjust after feeling one of my bra's straps slip off. She briefly paused to put on cosmetics as I got into her vehicle. No guy or woman would stand a chance when she made her entrance because of the vivid red lipstick and the top she was wearing.

"Andrea, I don't want you to assume that I'll have an appointment today. You may decide to bail out at the last minute and wait for me to finish inside the vehicle, if you so want. Unfortunately, it would have resulted in you wasting some valuable time without ever meeting her. However, Tina is unaware of your arrival, and I am certain that she will be alright. She likes me, therefore I'm certain that she'll like you too. It's not like our personalities are too different from one another. Anyone would want to be friends with us since we are kind ladies.

"I'm the same way, and I used to get compliments from my ex-boyfriends that I was a very energetic lady and a bit louder than others when it came to sex, ha ha. Even today, the way I scream in the middle of the night disturbs some people. You're correct, and I've listened to you, but I can't really do anything about it. We both understood that I was essentially a captive audience at the moment, I believe. Her laughter now made me realize that she was recalling something from when we were kids.

We had to pause there and stare at the lake and let out a collective sigh of happiness because the location was just as I remembered it.

I went over to Tina, who was standing right by the entrance, after telling Andrea that I would talk to her first.

"I notice you brought Kelly, your buddy. Was she the one who drove you here in the automobile the other day to see me? She looks a bit familiar to me. I caught a glimpse of her in the vehicle, and now that I get a closer look, I can fairly state that you both look lovely. I turned to greet her and gave her a hearty embrace to let her know I was glad to see her.

When I visited Andrea, she was totally transfixed by Tina's beauty and was unable to communicate or use any of her cognitive abilities. She said, "I would say from her reaction that you told how I helped you to relax so much the other day." When Tina approached her, she grabbed her hand and kissed the back of it with her tongue.

"Oh my... It feels good, ha ha.

"If you agree that it feels good, remain and talk to my buddy, who is also learning massage techniques. She is a fellow student massage therapist named Tia. She now visits me approximately three times each week after we became close. Come along, and I'll show you who she is. I was close behind her as she pulled Andrea into the home by the hand. Andrea could have simply promised to wait until I completed my visit, but she didn't even make an attempt. She was trailing after the serene vibe that was emanating from Tina and the white massage suit that was just partially closed. She had visible breast swell, and I could see the shadow of her mound, which I had already been quite used to.

When I arrived, they were both standing at the foot of the bed of a small Asian girl who was laying there with her eyes closed and her whole body on show. They had gone up the stairs. She was really attractive as she lay on the blankets, a sheen of perspiration clinging to her skin.

"I believe that to get her going this morning, my buddy needs a really special massage. Why don't you provide a hand to me? Since Tia was still sleeping, we all almost laughed, but we restrained ourselves since it would not be as enjoyable to wake her up this way.

When Tina undid her top to show a magnificent black bra, she complained that it was very hot inside. Andrea audibly gasped in amazement and awe. When Tina turned to face Andrea after hearing this, she expressed her gratitude for coming today. She seems interested and pleased that she may also get an appointment.

"Well, you remind me a lot of Kelly. So attractive without even realizing it. She was unquestionably under Tina's hypnotic influence, and she was using it to lull Andrea to sleep. Your physique is amazing, and those hips need to be classified as a deadly weapon, ha ha. I saw as August soaked in the praises before focusing her gaze on her attractive face and her beautiful, black hair.

"I know you're here because Kelly told you about how I use nice techniques that really help a woman have the relaxation she deserves, and I love that this is what I do all day long," the speaker said.

"Tina, August has never had a massage before and is a little hesitant and reserved. By the way her face was acting, I assumed she was tense. When Andrea was not looking, Tina gave me a sidelong glance and licked her lips in a seductive manner. I felt a rush of desire. She approached me and lightly massaged my shoulder blades with her hands. I was groaning at the mere touch of her hands, a particular arousal coming from knowing what was about to happen.

"You brought a small treat, and I've been waiting for you to return. How kind of you, and maybe you'd want to study massage with my buddy Tia? She took both of my hands and pulled me over to a wood-grain dresser where she showed me a variety of oils. After circling each one with her finger, she picked up this white tube. "This one warms up when it comes into contact with human skin." She squirted the transparent liquid into my hands before slamming them together and rubbing them together till I felt that distinct warmth in my palm. Andrea was perplexed as she grabbed my wrists and pushed me down, where I ended up touching the girl's upper chest.

"AHHHHHH." I was addicted to the sound; it was almost like an aphrodisiac. I watched as she writhed on the bed, half sleeping and moaning, and I moved my hands across her shoulders and upper chest. "More...PLEASE...MORE" It was still going to come as a surprise to her when she realized she wasn't alone even if she may have assumed Tina was teaching her a technique since she wasn't opening her eyes.

She wants more, you heard her, so." She was first startled when her eyes opened at the suggestion, but she quickly cracked a cheerful grin and started to stretch her limbs to get out of bed.

My gaze focused on the ethereal emerald pools of this Asian temptress as I heard the bed move. Tia was a stunning exotic Asian woman who appeared too beautiful to be true. Tina was requesting my Andrea to take off some clothes so she could have a massage as she was seated on the opposite side of the bed. It was almost like a green signal for Tina to begin stroking her shoulders once she was down to her underpants. This time, she rolled over onto the bed and positioned her next to her while she was wearing those stunning, sensual undergarments.

"I believe you ought to change." She acted precisely as she was instructed, almost as if getting a massage usually went this way, which wasn't really the case. I assume you want the same level of relaxation I provided her, therefore I want to offer it to you as well. As she started to drip the oils, she was whispering in her ear. Her hands started massaging her muscles. She took a handful of needles and started inserting them into different areas of her body. She uttered this type of delightful sigh with each one that was entered, and then her legs parted to the side, allowing Tina better access.

"I don't know who you are, but if I had to make a guess, I'd assume you're close to Kelly. Kelly did inform me that her closest friend had told her about you, and that your description was inaccurate. They should be left alone, and they seem to be engrossed in their own small universe. Let me demonstrate my manual dexterity for you. Andrea seemed to be enjoying the time of her life and completely unaware of the relaxation taking on around her.

I kept looking at Tia as she swayed from side to side, and my eyes followed the movement of her cheeks.

"Tina informed me of your situation, and I'm happy that she was able to assist you. She really enjoys providing some comfort to women. She sometimes oversteps the mark because of her eagerness to please others and her good intentions, but she just wants to make others feel good. I assumed she was exaggerating, but you truly do have a great appearance. Simply said, do you melt in my tongue or in my hand? I giggled girlishly instead of responding with words. We moved into the other room so we could enjoy some peace and quiet. In fact, there was a candle on a table next to the massage table. She patted it, and I heard a sound, which caused me to look up to see what was going on and if Andrea was okay.

"From the sound of it, I would guess that Tina and Andrea were conversing and getting to know one another better. I don't see any reason why we couldn't if they can do that. She took a long time to pull down my garments as she assisted me in pulling them off.

"I see that someone is missing their underpants, and I've always thought that going commando was the best course of action. Bras make me feel so constrained, so if you don't need to wear one, don't. We had similar viewpoints, and I really wanted to raise her and encircle her waist with her little, adorable form. I found myself doing just that before setting her back down on her feet.

I'm sorry, but I had no choice.

Kelly, there is nothing to apologize for. Although it felt wonderful, I think you still have a session to finish. I'm not boasting when I say that after all my practice, I'm just as skilled as Tina. We both gained a great deal from one another, and I just recently discovered that she uses some very fantastic methods that you have personally experienced. I wasn't sure what to make of it, but then I understood that all of her customers sought her out because of the way she looked at a body differently. She did confide in me that your physique was exquisite, and after seeing it for myself, I wholeheartedly agree.

attraction and resentment

The females are allowed to enter the yurt before Bo unlocks the entrance. The girls leap into the floor bed in good fun and embrace. Bo unzips his shirt and lies down next to them. Alongside the bed, he lights some candles and switches on some music. He adds, "I'm so glad you beautiful ladies are here," as they are all lit up. He strokes his hands over the bodies of the females while they kiss. He strips off their clothing before removing his shorts. Giselle is sitting on Tamara's face as she is on her back. After donning a condom, he enters Tamara and grips Giselle's breasts. After having sex with each of them, they collapse into a nude heap and pass out. Giselle explains, "As long as we use protection, this is harmless fun." And he adds, "exactly." Tamara exclaims, "That was incredible."

They both nod off, and Tamara is the first to awaken in the morning. She uses the bong to take a hit in an effort to get over her hangover. She exits the building while wearing a dress and a sweater to use the restroom. She smiles as she scans the area, admiring the dew on the morning mist. She feels at home since the area is peaceful. As she enters the yurt again, she observes Tamara and Bo fighting. She feels a jealously pang as they engage in sexual activity. She gets some granola and coconut milk and returns to the fire after wondering about the other males in the community. George, one of the lads, is eating there by the fire. He gives her a grin. Tamara takes a seat next to him since she finds him to be quite appealing. "How's it going?" he asks.

So delicious, she says. I adore this place. "You want to try some of this omelette?" he asks. She responds, "Sure." He uses his fork to feed her. "Wanna see my place?" he asks with a grin. She responds, "Sure." He stands up, luring her with his towering figure. He is older than Bo and stronger. His home is spotless, and incense is burning. She comments, "Wow, you really keep your place nice." I enjoy cleanliness and structure, he claims. His home is furnished with exquisitely carved wood pieces, and all of his shelves are beautifully arranged. In his kitchen, there are shelves of food. She comments, "Wow, you're stocked up." He claims, "I make this furniture, and I sell it so I can afford to eat well." The woman remarks, "Wow, your furniture is really nice." "Thanks," he says. You know, I didn't want to sell narcotics like the others around here. It's safer to engage in lawful activity. Her comment is, "Good point." "Would you like some pancakes?" he asks as he sits at the kitchen table. She enthuses, "That sounds amazing!" "Coffee?" He queries. Oh yeah, this is great, she exclaims. I'm visiting you more often. You may come here whenever you want, he adds. He starts the kettle while getting down on one knee in front of her and lowering her dress. "Are you okay?" He asks as he approaches her with his head.

She grins while shaking her head no. Within her legs, he kisses her. She has a desire for George in place of her jealousy. She feels at ease with him and confident in his ability to look after her. He cooks for her after she gets off. Even his yurt is heated by a wood burner. She lies in his bed till midday, when the celebration outside begins, since she feels like hanging out with him. He encircles her as they exit the yurt and approach the fire, where everyone is already sipping homemade beer and sharing blunts. "Hey George, do you think we should plant corn now or is it too late?" asks Bo. "Hmmmm, I'd choose ground crops that don't require as much water and sunlight," George muses. I assume tomatoes since they grow quickly, along with kale, potatoes, squash, carrots, and cucumbers. Bo looks bewildered at Tamara as he discovers George is still holding her by the arm.

"Want to go take a shower?" asks Tamara as she takes a seat next to Giselle. Tamara has a lot of energy. Giselle responds, "Hell yes." They go to the outdoor shower area, which features gravity flow and rainwater collection. They laugh while washing each other. Tamara declares, "I'm so high." "Right," answers Giselle. I am not sure about my name. They smile while gazing up at the sky. You should view George's property, Tamara advises. There is a woodstove and a ton of food there. It is stunning. "Did you fuck him?" asks Giselle. Tamara explains, "He ate me out." Nice, Giselle says. Bo could, however, start acting strangely. I saw his gaze onto you. Giselle reaches out and grabs Tamara, saying, "Ooh you're so hot." They have sex.

The clouds in the sky are becoming darker as they return to the fire. Bo predicts that it will rain. Good time of day to visit the barn. When it's raining, we all congregate there. They travel to the barn after packing food and wine. There is a large party going on with around thirty people. There is a beautiful atmosphere in the space as the rain begins to fall on the barn's tin roof. Everyone relaxes thanks to the incense scent and the groovy music. Everyone in the audience is cheerful and youthful. People are quite kind and down to earth. While playing guitar and bongos, people are passing around blunts. A fire is burning in the barn's fireplace, and several guests go to the loft to exchange life experiences.

Bo talks about his experiences and how their growth season works. He claims that the crops are experiencing problems with white mold and an invading insect that he has seen on them. "I use a special mixture with water and put it on the plants for white mold," a different person from the neighboring town explains. They exchange gardening advice, and the girls list the things they need to pick up the next day in town. George isn't hitting on any other females, but Tamara is becoming more and more drawn to him. His arms are folded as he sits in the corner, grinning and mingling with passersby. She believes he is wise and that she could depend on him. "You want to go to town with us tomorrow?" she asks as she walks up to him. Sure, he responds. I have a few items I need to pick up. She adds, "cool." She senses something as he gives her his first kiss on the lips. He gives her a gentle kiss as they continue to cuddle and gaze into one other's eyes.

He claims, "There's something different about you." She chews her lips as she studies him. "Sleepover tonight?" she asks. "My pancakes are pretty good, huh?" he asks, grinning at her. She grinned and began to dancing. As she dances with her, Giselle approaches. Hey, I feel like you're paying him more attention than I am, she adds. George is now out of earshot. Tamara declares, "I'm fucking broke." Only he has any money in this place. We must get along well with him. Batteries, tampons, shampoo, soap, and other necessities are needed, for example. We should find a means to generate money, Giselle argues. I'm also in debt. I should definitely save the roughly $20 I have left over for petrol. Let's stay with George tonight, suggests Tamara, before Bo becomes used to our presence. Giselle flinches and exclaims, "Yikes."

Tamara explains, "I mean, we have nothing, and Bo is a pothead who is also broke." Giselle utters the words "shhhh here he comes." He dances while giving each of them a screwdriver drink. He envelops them in his arms as they grinned. He declares, "You are two of the most beautiful women I've ever seen." I need to go potty, Tamara says as she slides out from under his arm. She feels like leaving. As she enters the barn's composting toilet, she starts to feel pressure building. She inhales deeply and feels the booze calming her anxiety. She leaves again and reclines on the sofa covered by a blanket. She nods out, and Tamara quickly locates her and joins her in bed, much like two cats on a sofa. They don't often drink as much throughout the day.

After a little while, the rain stops, and people begin to collect their belongings in preparation for the trip back to their hamlet. Giselle is awakened by Tamara, and together they return through the muck with lanterns. On his porch, George is smoking. He says, "Come on in, ladies." Before entering George's home, they wash their feet before going there. He prepares them spaghetti, and they like how welcoming his home is. Take the bed, he orders the women. They get the impression that he is watching out for them and guarding them in some way. You have to be cautious with Bo, he adds as he sits down on his futon. He has sensitivity. The girls nod as they devour their spaghetti. They doze off on George's bed, while he dozes off on his futon.

They get up before dawn and prepare to go for town. The ladies borrow some clothing from Bo, who is sound asleep in his bed and oblivious to their entrance. They cram themselves into the pickup vehicle while sporting helmets and fleeces. When they arrive in the little town, they explore the store's meager selection of items. "Hey George, will you buy us some food?" Tamara asks. She thinks he would do anything for them because of her outgoing nature. Sure, he responds. I'll be pleased to. What more do you require? Just some toiletries, Giselle says. "Wine?" he asks. Tamara grins and adds, "You read my mind." They stock up on food, and the girls use the limited signal to contact their parents. They reassure their parents that everything is well and that their internships are fun. What happens when someone is injured, asks Tamara? Has it ever occurred, I mean? George explains, "It does. Even though I am familiar with basic first aid, nobody has health insurance. You are aware of the danger. Guys, I believe I'm becoming ill, Giselle says. My throat hurts so much. "Open your mouth, let me see," George urges. She utters "ahh" while sticking her tongue out.

"Yup, it seems that you have an infection. I won't drink to you, young woman. She expresses sadness and adds, "Man, swallowing hurts." They return to camp after getting her some throat spray. Bo ignores them as they approach with their bags of belongings. Bo, Tamara says "hi." Thank you for asking if I needed anything, he adds while continuing to prepare food without looking up. "You were passed out cold," she says. "Did you even try to wake me up?" he asks. She apologizes. She believes it's because she and Giselle remained with George that he still doesn't look at her. You ok?" she enquires. Just strive to be more compassionate, he advises. We rely on one another and support one another. Giselle remarks, "That was unkind." Man, I'm sorry. You two will have to start contributing on your own in this place, he adds. This isn't simply a day of nonstop partying.

Giselle replies, "I'm happy to." He continues, "Last time I gave you stuff to do in the garden, you got drunk and only did a little bit, so I had to finish up your shitty jobs." Hey, I'm sorry, Giselle says. I think I wasn't paying attention since I was having too much fun. You can't simply eat everyone's food, drink everyone's wine, and smoke everyone's marijuana and not participate, he sneers, adding, "Well try harder." She feels his voice rising as his jealousy begins to bubble up. "All right, guy, I apologized. I'll pitch in, okay? Listen, is this about George? she asks as she places her hand on his arm. Nothing took place. "Yeah right," he responds without raising his head. "His place is warm, and he made us food," Giselle exclaims. He didn't touch me, and I can't say for Tamara. He provided the bed and used the futon to sleep.

Listen, it's not about that, and I know you're probably lying anyway, Bo adds as he turns to face her. You you aware of how many careless hippie girls like you come to our area and put in zero hours of actual work? I had hoped you would be unique. She responds, "Calm down, guy. Just remain calm. She approaches the garden and observes it. "You want me to pull those weeds?" she asks. You don't know what is weeds and what isn't, he sighs. I must instruct you. If I don't instruct you to do anything, don't touch the garden. I don't need you to be a piece of sh*t.

When George approaches, he asks, "What's going on?" He speaks in a reassuring manner.

I eventually had to open my eyes, paddle carefully back to the side, and hunt for the bar because I had to get a drink. In the most incredible manner, I was dazed. Instead of the bar, I now noticed the beachside blonde relaxing on one of the sun loungers near the pool. This time, I could see every inch of her. She was far more attractive than I had thought she was at the beach, in my opinion. Not even close to doing her justice, she was stunning!

If I had been concerned that I could have been seen earlier giggling at her, I needn't have bothered. She was clearly looking at me, and I could tell by the expression in her eyes that she was taking in the scenery.

Danny

Although having a good time in the water, I determined that I must have the appearance of a crazy mermaid without any friends.

I would have enjoyed some companionship and a long, cool drink. I got out of the water with a paddle and went to get my towel. Unfortunately, the stunning brunette who had been standing on the beach was nowhere to be seen, so I wiped myself before collecting my belongings.

I came up with a hazy idea as I made my way back to my resort since I had no one else to satisfy for the remainder of the day. I could either go to one of the larger beaches and locate a bar there, or I could use the hotel pool's facilities. My decision to visit the pool was driven by the really amazing peek I received the day before.

The hotel was a part of a larger complex that also included a few independent villas. The complex's manicured pool area was surrounded by palm trees and several sizable jardinières that featured colorful geraniums and other plants.

I waited in a little line at the bar and ordered a long white rum, coconut, and lime cocktail. I then carried my drink to a sun lounger, the ice clinking against the glass. I topped up my sunblock since the sun was strong and I was worried about being overheated. I then took several slow sips of my beverage. I adjusted my sun lounger and made the decision to take a little nap.

I may have been startled out of my light sleep by a pair of neighboring tourists' unexpected, fun chuckles. A light breeze drifted over the pool as I sat up and took a few swallows of my beverage, licking my lips and wondered where I might get something to eat.

I was daydreaming about grilled chicken when I saw a girl's figure floating in the water on one of those inflatable toys. My thoughts briefly returned to the brunette on the beach. She had the same gorgeous tanned skin and luxurious black hair. I sat there admiring her flawless, lightly tanned figure as she drifted on the water, sometimes having swimmers' wakes disrupt her body. She did, in fact, sit up as I was watching and started to walk up to the edge of the pool. Since I could always recall her having such heavenly looks, I was certain it was her. She was breathtakingly lovely and was facing me.

Katie

I had been daydreaming about the blonde all day, thinking about how beautiful and seductive she was and how I would want to kiss and touch her in the most sensual manner. The pleasant surprise of seeing her at the pool was really appreciated. I threw caution to the wind and put on a "show" since I was so certain that she had been gazing at me while I was on the lilo. I did this to see how she would respond.

With my legs still partly spread out and draped over the lilo, I paddled my hands in little circles as I approached the pool's edge to align it properly in her direction. I jumped off it as dramatically as I could, throwing my leg over in a broad and high arc to give her the best possible view of all my goods. I couldn't help but grin at her since it felt so wicked.

I approached her sun lounger's end as I made my way over to the bar to fetch a beverage. I purposely swung my hips and pushed my boobs out as I passed, hoping without hope that she was still glancing my way. More than that, I really hoped she would approve of what she saw!

When I got to the bar, I posed as provocatively as I could while placing my drink order, sometimes casting a mischievous glance at the blonde. Her eyes were still fixed on me, which made me happy, and it just made me grin at her even more.

I urgently considered how to start a conversation while the waiter made me a pina colada. I made the decision to relax with my drink on the sun lounger next to hers and see what transpired.

I attempted to maintain my seductive display as I went across the terrace in the same manner as I had gone to the bar: all hips, bum, and boobs. My idea was ruined a few seconds later. My right foot accidentally brushed against the edge of the metal ladder going into the deep end of the pool because I was so focused on my stupid effort to seem attractive.

I fell forward awkwardly and landed at the edge of her lounger. The stumble wasn't that bad, but my drink flew out of my hand. The glass looped up, whirling as it flew, just missing her head before landing with a dull thud behind where she was sitting in a geranium pot. Pina colada wasn't as fortunate. She was covered in sticky goo that spilled out of the glass and down her front!

I wasn't sure whether to weep or laugh. She appeared even more stunning than before, with her perky nipples now sexily revealed through the soaking wet material of her bikini. She was also horrified when I essentially threw my drink all over her.

I was only able to blurt forth what undoubtedly came across as a bunch of rambling and incoherence.

God, oh God! I am very sorry. How am I supposed to make it up to you? My name is Katie, by the way. Hello!"

Danny

If the mystery girl had been staying at my hotel, it would have been a wonderful coincidence, but as her little blow-up lilo whirled on the water, I was certain it was the girl from the beach. She was beautiful from every aspect, and I watched her shamelessly as she started paddling towards the pool's edge. She looked stunning in her red bikini. I could see the bow near her hip, and I tried to picture how I would remove the bottom part of it by grabbing it in my teeth.

She was clearly gazing my way and I could see that she wanted to leave the pool, but I only recognized this through the fog of my fantasy. Her "coming ashore" was done in a different way. She raised her leg off the lilo and rotated in such a manner that I had a really great glimpse of her special area. It was a genuine performance. In a less public setting, I may have been less discreet as a tingling of joy caused me to wiggle in my chair.

She eventually emerged from the water, moved toward me, then made a sharp turn to face the bar on my left. She was in close proximity to me for the first time. She had the most lovely buttocks I had recently seen, along with a well toned figure, huge boobs, and she was nothing short of breathtaking. She walked in a sensual manner that caused her hair and butt to swing. She stopped at the bar, casually glanced in my direction, and gave me a gorgeous grin, which I responded. If the pool-walking incident wasn't overt flirting, that grin most surely was. I chewed my lip in anticipation of what would come next. She might have wiggled away, leaving me to wonder, or she could have moved.

I didn't have to wait long since after serving me, she came back over to where I was sitting near the edge of the pool. I didn't try to disguise my fascination with and hunger for her delectable figure. She had a drink in her hand and was staring at me, but she was standing too near to the pool's edge. She tripped over something as she turned to move toward me, creating an absurd situation that almost bordered on comedy as her drink flew across the room and she made a little squeak. Her drink spilled all over me while I waited for the sound of shattering glass, leaving me momentarily cold but sticky, and she fell to the ground in a heap.

To my delight, she was unharmed, stood up, and introduced herself as Katie in the loveliest manner imaginable. If it had been anybody else, I would have laughed out loud.

I said, "Hey, I'm Danny." Saying "Thanks for the drink!"

I licked the tip of my finger after running it over my abdomen.

A "Pina Colada?"

She bowed.

Saying "I'm so sorry!"

No damage was done. It is a little sticky, however, and I could dry out strange.

"...Yes?"

As I said, I fixed my gaze on her stunning brown eyes. You may return to my room and assist me in tidying up.

Three: The Shower

Katie

Embarrassment caused my face to become crimson red, although it didn't stay long. She was very beautiful, and Danny clearly had a humorous and carefree personality to match. The fact that we were now conversing made me laugh since I had felt foolish after my fall and for spilling my drink all over her.

Even better than that, Danny had just asked me to assist in cleaning her up in her room. That was an invitation I would never decline, I tell you!

I smiled and said, "I'd love to. To help her get off the couch, I reached out with my hand. "Lead the way, then."

Danny grasped my fingers tightly and dragged me away down the hallway to the rooms.

I grinned at her and replied, "Well, I think there are two ways I could clean you up," after we had entered her room and closed the door behind us.

She said, "Oh, and what did you have in mind for each of those?"

I answered, "It would be simpler for me to show you than to tell you about them."

"Okay. What comes first? Danny queried.

I replied, "Umm...this," before leaning in and giving her a little kiss on the lips. Danny gave back the kiss without thinking twice. She drew me in by connecting the fingers of both of her hands with mine. Before giving her another, much deeper kiss than the first, I stroked the tip of my tongue over her lips.

When Danny finally broke the kiss, he continued, "But that bit wasn't dirty, Katie," and he winked at me with a humorous expression.

I said, bending against her neck and kissing some of the sticky pina colada off her skin, "I know....but this bit is,"

I could feel goosebumps beginning to form on her arms and chest as my tongue stroked around her neck, and I knew Danny was loving the way I was helping to clean her up. I was inspired to take further risks by her response. And this part also has to be cleaned, I added.

I kissed her over the top hem of her bikini bottoms as I knelt down and stroked my tongue across her still-wet stomach. I could see pina-colada rivulets still gently flowing from the wet cloth down her legs. I bent down in front of her and kissed and licked Danny's front thighs. My hands moved up and down the backs of her legs while my tongue followed the rivulets everywhere they went.

I made my way gently back up Danny's body, using my tongue to lick and caress the now-sticky residues of my drink. Before loosening the bow on the back of her bikini top and slipping the straps off her shoulders, my fingertips gave her a little scratch along the spine. Her nipples were still perky from their wetting, and her breasts slipped free of the wet cloth. I leaned forward and kissed each nipple in turn, circling each areola with the tip of my tongue. I gently sucked on Danny's now-erect nipples while relishing the flavor of my drink as I pulled and nibbled her nipples between my lips, rolling them back and forth.

"There. As I rose to my feet in front of her, I remarked, "That's a wonderful start to having you all straightened out. Here is a second approach.

Once again holding Danny's hand, I escorted her to the restroom.

"We're taking a shower now!" I said.

The Desert Eagle semi-automatic handgun made an unbearable noise. But it is what you anticipate at a shooting range.

Emma saw that she had hit the dummy human in the centre of his chest as she turned to face him at the other end of the shooting range.

"Hey, can I have a minute of your time?" Emma did not hear the girl who had just entered through the door, and shot another bullet, that would have pierced the skull of an actual human target.

"Emma?" The girl spoke a little loudly this time.

When Emma looked around, the beauty in front of her caught her attention.

Lily was younger and had a more athletic figure than Emma, who was shorter but had a curvier frame. Her cat-like eyes radiated sensuality, her cheekbones were prominent, and her jet-black hair fell straight beyond her shoulders.

If Kendall Jenner had been dressed in a police uniform and walked down the runway, the girl would have resembled Kendall Jenner.

"Hello, I missed seeing you there. These locations have very loud noise. How may I be of service to you? You aren't around here anymore, have you?

"I am new, yes. I have been moved from the Charleston precinct. My buddy was killed during a firefight. So they moved me here and put me under your wing. I so decided to stop by and say hello.

Emma gave the girl a brief moment of attention. checking every inch of her new hire.

"That is awful to hear, I'm sorry. Yes, Steve did inform me that I would have a fresh female assigned to me; but, I had anticipated a recent academy graduate rather than someone who has previously been seen about this dishonest city. Tell me your name.

Lilian Collins. Well, I just recently graduated. We got into a gunfight at a bar on my third day on patrol, Lily said, her expression clearly troubled by the memories.

For the girl in front of her, Emma felt horrible. She could see the pain in her eyes, but she also couldn't help but comment on how lovely they were.

How could a young lady like her become a police officer? She ought to be strutting the runways and enticing men and women with her long legs and toned physique.

On the third day of your work, a shootout? Given that they don't assign newly hired soldiers to monitor particularly volatile regions, that is unusual. For them to put their faith in you with a location like Charleston, you must have excelled in the academy. Emma threw the pistol on a nearby table, took off her headphones, and untied her ponytail as she added, "I mean, I can tell you are in better condition than 90% of the ladies who are recruited in the force.

Lily was astounded by her senior's beauty. Emma's fearlessness and

73

badassness had already been described to her by everyone, but no one had informed her that Emma herself looked like Shakira.

Lily had brown eyes and blonde hair that was curled. Her figure had an hourglass shape, and her lips were large and luscious. She had a little tattoo of a Phoenix rising toward her earlobe on the side of her neck.

"Since I graduated at the top of my class, people assumed that the daughter doesn't need a lot of child care. Lily pointed to the rifle and remarked, "I see that you are quite excellent at that.

Years of practice make you like that. Well, if I'm being honest, it wasn't simply practice. These abilities were also often required of me in the outside world. I've been in your position many times before. More lovers have passed away than I care to recall.

The question is, "How long have you been a policewoman?"

"15 years. I was sworn in when I was 21, so I'm assuming that's also your age.

"I am 21, yes. However, you don't seem 36. I mean, when I first saw you, I assumed you were in your late 20s," stated Lily.

Emma grinned and looked Lily in the eyes. "Thanks, I suppose. Look at you, however. You don't even resemble a police officer. You seem to have hurt a few dozen people simply getting to the police station.

At her first encounter with her partner and senior, Lily flushed, something she truly did not want to do.

Can I give it a go? asked Lily as she pointed at the weapon.

Naturally, I'd want to see what the student who placed first in her class can do.

Lily giggled, "Thank you for the extra pressure.

"Don't worry; if you behave badly, I won't tell anybody. I'll keep your secret secure, said Emma.

After counting the number of rounds left in the cartridge, Lily took up the Desert Eagle and glanced at Emma before adding, "But you will know, and I really want to impress you."

Emma was watching Lily from behind as she took aim.

Lily caught Emma's attention as she admired her tall, lean form. She could easily see Lily's adorable and petite ass, its delicate curve clearly discernible in the form-fitting police pants Lily was sporting.

This chick seems problematic. Delicious difficulty.

Bang, Bang, and BANG.

Three consecutive headshots.

Lily gave Emma a wink as she tilted her head to gaze at her.

Emma had a stomach-dropping sensation.

Bang, Bang, and BANG.

Three more headshots.

Lily made her way back to where Emma was standing and did the same thing Emma did by throwing the pistol onto the table.

Am I okay? Lily queried.

Emma's face abruptly lost all expression and her smile vanished.

Very good. These are just the fundamentals. A girl at the top of her class ought to have at least done this much, in my opinion. However, I will offer it to you since you deserve it.

Emma's face regained its grin.

"Thanks, manager. So tomorrow will be our first patrol, am I correct?

Don't call me your boss, first of all. Your companion, I am.

But because you exude such powerful, alpha emotions, I feel compelled to give you a suitable moniker. How awful is it really?

"All good, give me any call you want. And yeah, tomorrow is the day of our first patrol. However, I don't like to start my patrol from the police station. Meet me down the street at Harry's Diner. It is in plain sight. Although it has the worst appearance of any restaurant you will ever see, its waffles are incredible.

I have no surgical issues. However, I shall keep you company," Lily said, leaning her head to the side and flashing

Emma one of the prettiest grins she had ever seen.

I'm going to die because of this girl.

Emma questioned, "What do you have for breakfast then?"

"Sandwich with avocado and salad."

Emma rolled her eyes and said, "Millennials," "Okay, I'll see you tomorrow, Lily," as she shook the girl's hand and felt the softness of her skin. She then felt something between Lily's legs.

***

The waffles were excellent as always. Emma was astounded by how underestimated certain places were simply because the proprietor lacked the funds to make the restaurant or diner seem upscale or contemporary. Perhaps appearances were more important than everything else.

But Lily had both.

She had ability and was gorgeous. She was nonetheless also tardy.

The door opened just as Emma was going to call her, and Lily entered while scanning the area for Emma.

Emma said, "Over here," and Lily sprinted over to her.

Their thighs were in contact when she sat next to Emma. A strange position for two coworkers to be in.

"I apologize sincerely for arriving late. You just finished eating your waffle, I notice.

It's OK. You weren't going to keep me company anyhow, right?

Although I wouldn't have eaten it, I would have enjoyed to just chat with you.

I don't talk much when I'm eating. So in the end, everything turned out just great," Emma added while wiping her mouth with a tissue.

Should we depart now? replied Emma.

"May I have some coffee? I was already so late that I was unable to have one.

"Sure," Emma said.

Lily needed a coffee, so Emma contacted the waiter she knew by name and placed the order.

"So, what caused your delay? partying outside? overindulged a little bit?" Looking out the restaurant window at the deserted streets that would gradually come to life as the morning went on, Emma smirked and inquired.

I never drink. I had invited my nephew to stay with me. I simply wanted to spend some time with him since I knew I would be quite busy starting today," said Lily.

Emma noticed a faint undertone of grief in Lily's voice as she turned to face her spouse.

Are you close to your nephew, then?

Yes, it's really near. He used to spend most of his time with me since his mother, my sister, died a few years ago, and his father is often gone on business. But I haven't been able to spend much time with him since I was initiated.

Lily, I'm very sad to hear that.

It's OK. Lily remarked, her lips curling into a grin but sorrow in her eyes. "It's been a long time since she passed away, and even though we mourn her a lot, we have grown stronger over the years.

"Listening to you talk about looking after and supporting your nephew has impressed me more than six headshots did. Lily, you are such a beautiful girl and a brave young woman. You must also have a partner in life, I'm sure of it.

Yes, Lily said as her coffee soon followed, "I have a partner, and we've been together for four years now. I believe I will most likely get hitched to this man. He has been really encouraging throughout all of my difficulties.

Lily said, "That is amazing to hear," but she also experienced some melancholy.

"How about you, manager? Who gets to tap that ass, the fortunate one? Lily apologized for the vulgarity, took a drink of coffee and arched one brow like Dwayne Johnson.

As single as they come, I am. This ass won't be tapped anytime soon. I've been in far too many unsuccessful relationships to begin another one right now. I only fuck random girls nowadays.

Lily almost spat up her coffee.

"I'm sorry, I didn't intend to respond that way. I was simply taken off guard by you.

"Really? What was more unexpected? The term "fuck" itself, or the fact that I "fuck" girls? Emma leaned back in her chair and inquired, casting a sidelong glance at Lily as she wiped coffee off her jeans.

"Both, in fact. Yet more strength to you. I had no idea the police department was accepting enough to employ lesbians.

"They are ignorant. They didn't know when I joined, but as time passed, they started to wonder. They were unable to terminate me because I had become so skilled at my work. Do you find it offensive that I'm gay?

"No, never, never. Actually, I adore it.

"Why? Do you also have an interest in women? Lily did her best not to look Emma in the eyes as she questioned her as she was fixedly looking at her.

I don't want to be disrespectful, I say.

Lily, I won't take offense. You are free to speak as you choose.

I had an awful experience in college, Lily replied after inhaling deeply. My sorority members attempted to push themselves on me, and they were successful. I haven't given it any more attention since then. Lily replied as she gulped down the last of her coffee, "I hope you get it.

"I perceive. But don't let a few of females represent our whole community.

Lily said, "Of course I don't," and grinned.

"Should we leave at this time?" Eva enquired.

Yes, do we need to travel anywhere or are we simply patrolling here?

"Don't worry, it's not the strip club where your partner was shot, but it sounds like a strip club in our neighborhood is also having the same issues as the one in Charleston. We're heading to a strip club. We must therefore go ask the strippers some questions in order to avoid any similar occurrences. Are you prepared?

I'm ready, boss, Lily exhaled after taking a long breath.

***

Lily and Emma entered a poorly lit room that had been transformed into a makeshift strip club with only one pole on a stage with inconsistent lighting and ancient, ripped leather seats that seemed to be invaded by animals from another planet.

Hey, there it is. Your favorite client, Stacy, is in the room. And look at the hot she brought along. When Emma entered the strip club, a red-haired dancer said, "Looks like you are in for a lit of work today, missy."

"I have come on duty, Sylvia, but don't worry, Stacy hasn't rid herself of me just yet," remarked Emma as she brushed by Sylvia, a stripper.

Lily followed Emma down the hallway, through a few ladies, some young and elderly men, and strippers who seemed to have been working the floor for a long time.

Emma paused to talk with a tall, blonde-haired lady, whispering something in her ear before moving on, not before giving the blonde a gentle squeeze on the behind.

Lily was only able to stand and stare in shock at what had just occurred, but once she had recovered herself, she followed Emma down a long corridor that led to a black wooden door at the end of the hallway.

Lily followed Emma's opening of the door.

They discovered a lady, who was formerly a stripper herself, seated behind a desk, seeming anxious and agitated, with puffy eyes and bandaged wrists in different locations.

As the two policewomen entered the room, the lady glanced up, and her eyes brightened up.

"I am overjoyed that you are here. I'm so relieved, oh my god, I can't even tell you," the stripper said excitedly.

"I see you. It seems like there are fights going on in a stripper wrestling league. Why the heck did it happen to you?

"Emma, how dare you make me laugh? "Look at me!"

Oh, girl, relax your titties. The first step to recovery is to laugh at yourself. Tell me, who attacked you; tell me now. Emma asked as she sat down across from the lady, and Lily joined her.

"The men of Richard Morrison. All of the strip clubs in this region have been experiencing issues because of them. I'm not sure what their issue is. In fact, it seems that they are biased against Jacob. Only the strippers who work with him appear to be the targets of their harassment. The lady spoke in an angry tone, her eyes wide, giving her inflated face an even stranger appearance.

Richard Morrison once more? I knew it would be him, but I had no idea that so soon after the other event I would have to hear his name from a stripper.

Is this the same Richard Morrison whose guys assassinated my partner? Lily interjected abruptly.

Emma sighed and said, "Never discuss a case in front of a victim, and yes, it is the same Richard Morrison, although we never seem to have enough evidence to ever arrest him."

Anyway, there was this Mark man who requested a personal lap dance. I could see right away that he was one of those macho, noisy sorts that believed they owned us just because they had paid for a lap dance. I then lead him into one of the private rooms, and we start. This guy was clearly being too helpful, as you know, Jacob has a severe rule against people being too handy during a lap dance," the lady said, waiting for the policewomen to say anything. When they didn't, she added, The stripper pointed to her face and stated, "I batted his hand away several times, but each time he continued becoming more forceful, and towards the end this occurred.

Why didn't you dial 911 at that point? Lily queried.

"It was too late; the manager on duty was unable to reach Jacob, therefore we were unable to go further without his consent. We still haven't filed a formal complaint. I assumed that Stacy's knowledge of a police officer who could assist us would be the best course of action. Given that Jacob is too weak to take any action.

"Laura, why do you suppose that is?" Eva enquired.

"I'm not sure. Undoubtedly, Richard Morrison frightens him. He is a strong guy.

For a few minutes, the room was silent.

Are you certain you don't want to file a formal complaint? Emma leaned closer and inquired, her golden wavy hair reflecting the sun as it reflected off her head.

"No, it would mean my employment would disappear. Just keep doing what you're doing and protect us more, please.

"You understand we can't do that. A place the government doesn't want to get involved with is a strip club. We also cannot launch an inquiry until you file a formal complaint.

What about the murder of my partner? Yes, the cops are looking into it. Lily turned to Emma with a heated face, "And if Richard's men were behind the shooting, this offers us a straight shot at him.

It's not that simple, however. I'll elaborate later. I want you to go home and relax for the time being, Laura. Emma added, gazing directly into Laura's eyes, "And if you truly want me to assist you, then I would want to ask you just one tiny favor.

"Yes?"

"Please give me Jacob's cell phone number," I said.

"Honey, stay a little while longer. I am aware of how demanding your work is. Stacy stopped Emma by holding her wrist and tugging her toward herself. "Let me take care of that stress for you," she said.

We must go on, Stacy. We've just started the day's patrol. You are aware that my weekends are yours. Stacy's left breast was softly cupped by Emma as she stated, "I've been missing these lovely things a lot.

"How about the fresh face? She has been looking at me nonstop. Will you, honey? I'm sure she'd want to try some of them as well.

Stacy's stunning tits caught Lily's attention, but she quickly diverted her look and feigned not to hear.

"Won't forcing her to do the rite be initiating her? She is without a doubt the sexiest woman you have ever taken to a bar. Stacy continued, this time speaking a bit louder, "And I would definitely like to run my hands all over her long legs and amazing body."

This time, Lily's curiosity won out.

"What kind of initiation?" As the stage stripper finished with her song and gathered the dollar containers scattered all around the dance floor, she inquired, turning back to look at Stacy.

"Oh, so she's unaware? Do you want for me to inform her? asked Stacy of Emma.

Emma glanced at Lily to assess the circumstance, then nodded her head as if she had already made up her mind. "Lily, as you must have seen, I am a very sexually open, upfront person who is also into women. As a kind of tradition, I need each lady who joins me as a companion to have a lap dance from the finest of the best here, Stacy. The ladies always finish up with Stacy here grinding on their laps and her tits in their mouths because they all want to impress me. Some of them ultimately do a bit more than that. But given what happened with you in college, I believe I can give you a pass," Emma added before returning to her conversation with Stacy.

After hearing what Emma had just said and hearing the 2pac song being played loudly over the speakers, Lily glanced at Emma and suddenly felt the need to show her that she was superior to any other female who had ever worked with her.

I'll carry it out, Lily replied.

Emma paused her conversation with Stacy and smiled broadly as she turned to see Lily.

"Really? Are you certain?

"No, but I must adhere to tradition if there is one. That is why I identify as a traditionalist.

Oh what a bunch of nonsense. Do you want to carry it out? You want to do it because you cannot be the girl who chose not to follow in the footsteps of others. My God! I have never seen a female as competitive as you. You know you make me think of myself. You want it, then?

Lily exhaled deeply and said, "Yes," turning to face Stacy.

She had to admit that Stacy was a stunning lady. Stacy was a total beauty and reminded Lily of supermodel Barbara Palvin because of her bright blue eyes, doll-like face, model-like figure, and larger breasts than the normal model.

"I must be fortunate today. I get to take your virgin lap dance? I must forewarn you that I could be a bit more nifty with you than usual. Your body is a cigarette! Emma, take a look at her face. She is very beautiful!"

Emma just stood and grinned, causing Lily to flush uncontrollably.

Emma looked at Lily while speaking to Stacy, "She is all yours, I guess," she said.

Stacy grabbed Lily's hand and motioned for her to follow her down the hallway to the private enclosures, where the actual action took place. "Follow me, hun, for the time of your life," she said.

Stacey placed Lily onto a couch after entering one of the private rooms and then leaned back against the wall for a few seconds to simply stare at Lily.

"You have never dated a female, correct?"

"Voluntarily? No."

If you do, I'll make sure you never date a male again after today.

"Highly unlikely."

Stacey responded, "Let's see," and then she drew closer to Lily, sitting on her lap.

She took Lily's hand in hers and led Lily's fingers to her lips, gently brushing them against Lily's lower lip. She then guided Lily's fingers to her face and brought them to her breasts, which were held up by a very sensual black lace bra. Finally, she made Lily gently press her boobs while continuing to gaze into Lily's brown eyes with her own blue ones.

As Lily's hands tightened around Stacy's tits, she suddenly felt a surge. She was unable to look away from Stacy's since, all of a sudden, the lady gained even more attractiveness.

Lily unclasped Stacy's bra on her own initiative when Stacey directed Lily's hands to her back.

Stacey murmured, "Bite the front of my bra and pull it down, babe," and Lily did it without thinking.

Being an alpha female outdoors, Lily found that obeying a stripper was really thrilling. Suddenly, all she wanted to do was follow this Barbara Palvin lookalike's instructions.

Her tongue lightly touched Stacy's nipple as she tugged Stacy's bra down, and she suddenly felt euphoric.

Lily lost control of her senses and gave in to urges she never imagined she possessed as Stacy ran her hands through her hair, untied her ponytail, and delicately kissed her forehead before slowly pressing Lily's face into her breast and simply keeping it there.

"What do you want to do right now, Lily?"

Kiss your breasts.

I believe you should first lick my nipples since they are begging for your attention.

Lily paused for a second before gently licking Stacy's nipple with her tongue.

It became difficult right away.

Lily then gave it many kisses in succession.

Then, while Lily continued kissing Stacy's breasts without being very assertive or forward, Stacy started pounding her ass against her thighs.

Even though she wanted to let out the horny monster within her, she couldn't because of her anxiety since this was still new ground for her.

Lily gave Stacy a tight embrace while around her waist.

Oh my, I just saw someone being sensual. Yes, keep stroking your nipples, and let me to smear your thighs with my pussy. You look so gorgeous, fuck. The fact that I will be compensated for something I am so loving is wrong.

Lily turned away from Stacy's nipple to gaze at the person sitting on her lap. She was in amazement. Suddenly, she recalled the episode from her time in college, and it all started to make sense.

Without averting her gaze from Stacy, Lily said, "Pull on my hair."

"What?"

Pull as much of my hair as you can, then kiss me. Better yet, bite me.

'I can't do that. There is no BDSM club here. Even though I can't kiss you, I did it anyhow since you are so lovely.

Pull my hair, then, for the same purpose. Lily pleaded with the listener, her face contorted into a miserable expression.

I beg you to spit on me. Just do it, you whore! Fuck you.

Stacy was attacked by Lily, who grabbed her hand and put it to her neck.

"Okay, then, just choke me. Look at what you did. You exposed suppressed aspirations. How come you did it? You must now appease me. "Crush me!"

Stacy had wide-open eyes. She was seeing a change that she could not have predicted. The police officer who had been so reserved and icy had abruptly changed.

And this individual was determined to achieve her goals at any costs.

She also wants to be humiliated and mistreated.

Stacy sat back down after rising off Lily's lap.

"Officer, the time is up. I believe you should go.

Lily remained still.

Her heart was thumping wildly inside of her as she glanced up at Stacy and then down at the ground. She was perspiring and the walls all around her were suddenly covered with ripples, as if they were just water's surface reflections.

"Are you okay?" Stacy inquired, suddenly in a panic.

"Emma? EMMA?"

Stacy shouted for the senior policewoman as she dashed outside.

***

The faint crackling of the radio broke the stillness in the vehicle.

Backup was already its route as a robbery was reported in the area.

Emma turned to face Lily, who was bathed in a strong red light emanating from the strip club's neon sign.

"How are you feeling right now?"

"Better."

Is it OK for me to ask you what transpired inside at this time?

"The incident's recollection brought on a panic attack. Even though I had anticipated this, I hadn't anticipated the intensity to be this high.

"You did really have a panic attack. This much was obvious. But it appeared like you were enjoying the lap dance a bit too much just before the panic episode. If you remembered anything, it didn't make you feel anxious or frightened, says Stacy; rather, it appeared to have turned you on even more.

Lily quickly turned her head to look at Emma while furrowing her brows in response to her question, "So you are saying that I am lying?"

"No, I'm just curious as to why you would ask someone to choke you, because if you had been sexually assaulted in the past, that is the last thing you would ask someone to do."

I don't know what that stripper told you, but that didn't happen, Lily said as she grinned and peered out the vehicle window. I didn't request that she choke me. That is just nonsense.

Are you certain? Emma said sternly.

"Yes, I'm positive."

"Okay, I'll do as you say. You ought to relax at home, in my opinion. With a spouse who isn't entirely well, I don't want to go out on the streets. I would be the one they would hold accountable if anything were to happen to you, Emma added as she started the vehicle.

I'm not ready to return home. Emma, this is my first day. I didn't have a major panic attack, therefore I don't want to hide and flee.

"Lily, I didn't ask you to go home. I'm giving you the go-home order. Do you like having things ordered of you? Lily heard something sneaky in Emma's tone as she said.

"Who told you that?" I asked.

"The stripper you believe to be fabricating stories. She may have made this up as well, isn't that right?

Lily remained silent. As the automobile sped forward, her eyes were fixated on the road in front of her.

***

Cross-legged and sitting on her bed in the dark, Lily was mentally recreating the episode from college. She had worked to bury the memories of that day for years, and she had been successful.

But now that Emma and her stripper buddy had managed to get beyond her barriers, she found herself, after a long period, slowly slipping back into the same pit from which she had previously emerged.

The last image she had in her head before going to sleep was of herself lying on a bed in her dorm room with four girls bending over her, her hands and legs bound to the frame, and a fifth girl ramming a huge, nine-inch dildo into her pussy as the other girls pulled on her nipple clamps, causing her pain-induced cries to turn into screams of pleasure.

As I got out of the taxi and gave the driver his tip, the rain cut the glass. I felt more terrified than ever as I watched the taxi leave.

A few individuals were waiting at the door of the club, handing the bouncer their ID cards as the neon sign of the club flashed before my eyes.

I wished I had left my ID at home.

I prayed I wasn't attractive enough to be permitted entry into the club, but alas, I know I am a lovely lady, and tonight, dressed in a skirt with a thigh-high slit and an off-shoulder blouse, I knew I was looking prettier than ever.

I took a deep breath and waited for the people in front of me to enter. It wasn't until I was standing on the sidewalk by myself, the wind roaring all around me and making my overcoat flap like a flag on a pole, that I decided to approach the enormous, balding guy with arms that seemed to be strong enough to uproot a tree.

I introduced myself and asked to join the club, and the guy gave me a weird look.

"I've never heard it expressed that way before. Please show me your ID.

I gave the guy my ID before taking a quick, uneasy check around.

There were no cars on the highways, and the only windows in the buildings that bordered the narrow lane where the club was located had lights on; the other windows were completely black.

To be very honest, I would have also allowed you to enter without the ID. If you know what I mean, the club isn't a very pleasant place to be tonight if you're a lad.

Despite not understanding what the guy was saying, I nodded and attempted to smile at him.

"You are prepared. Welcome to Club Sin City, Madame," the guy said as he moved to the side and unlocked the club's big wooden entrance.

The powerful bass of speakers playing a strongly autotuned rap song assaulted me as soon as the door was opened.

The guy locked the door behind me as I entered the club.

My breathing was labored, and I felt like I may pass out right there.

But nevertheless I managed to remain composed.

You must constantly make intentional attempts to venture outside of your comfort zone if you want to change your life or break out of the rut you're in.

The club's decor matched my expectations to a tee. It wasn't that I had never gone to a club; rather, it had been a while since my previous visit, and even then, I had Steve at my side, so I didn't have to worry about anything.

The walls were decorated with additional neon lights and multicolored lasers reflected off of them as they flashed to the rhythm of the music.

A giant overhead spotlight lit the dance floor, where individuals of different shapes, sizes, and tastes were dancing together. Some seemed as though they had done this before, while others appeared to be hearing music for the first time and unclear of how one should move their bodies.

I recalled my most recent club experience. That night, it rained as well, and I was wearing a body-hugging dress that highlighted my considerable curves. Steve kept his hand on my bottom the whole time, refusing to let it even after we stopped dancing.

I suddenly felt like I had been hit in the face by the idea of Steve. Realizing that this is often how my descent into sadness starts, I knew I needed to keep my composure tonight.

Tonight was meant to be a night of beginning over.

Even while leaving despair behind and letting go of Steve's memories is a move that first appears incredibly thrilling, once we really do it, we understand how difficult the trip will be.

I shook my head in an attempt to get my thoughts of Steve to exit through my ears, but all it did was pain my head.

I was aware of my needs. Whiskey.

I eventually became aware that people were looking at me as I crossed the club to go to the bar, which was beyond the dance floor.

The majority of those looks belonged to males, but I also saw a few glances from women, as if my sheer presence in the club threatened their authority.

I was used to women competing with me and criticizing me based simply on my beauty before they ever had a chance to talk to me.

I was taller than most models, but I had thicker legs and an ass. Because of my Persian ancestry, many thought I looked exotic, and my broad, thick lips and my large, brown eyes—which, in my opinion, were my greatest feature— added to those exotic qualities.

But if you had asked Steve, he would have told you right away that my legs were the best feature of my body because he preferred tall women, and the last woman he cheated on me was the same height as me. Later, when I learned the names of the girls he had been seeing behind my back, I realized that Steve preferred tall girls with big eyes.

When I eventually caught Steve jerking off to Mahlagha Jaberi's Instagram photographs, I understood he wasn't kidding when he would often say how similar the two of us looked and compare me to the Persian model.

But all of that had already happened, when I had been betrayed by a guy who had been my boyhood darling, and I had once again allowed myself to be carried away by ideas of the devil.

While waiting for my drink, I turned around once again to gaze at the club after ordering a 30ml glass of Jack Daniels.

The already busy space was still being filled around ten o'clock at night.

What would be my next move, I pondered.

How long was my resolve going to hold? I had managed to get myself inside the club, ordered a drink, and resisted the impulse to rush outside into the rain, get a taxi, and hide in the warmth of my bed.

A female squeaked in between me and a guy who was busy flirting with a lady who was obviously out of her league while I was thinking these things in my brain.

I was not immediately aware that the girl was not alone.

The pair was now groaning next to me while resting on the bar counter, and the bartender was waiting for them to finish before taking their order. She was eating the face of another female.

The girl who was having her face chewed said, "Babe...babe...we have to order," but she was unable to stop herself.

The fact that two females were kissing in front of me for the first time despite my best efforts to avoid doing so.

I was curious and eager to learn more.

I sat down at the bar with my elbows propped up, turned to face it, and glanced at the pair as they continued to embrace passionately.

The girl who wanted to place the drink order was a short brunette with a fringed bob hairstyle, thick eye makeup, and flared pants that gave her a very affluent look. She also wore a jacket without a shirt inside.

I was drawn to the other girl, however.

I questioned if I would ever be able to pull off anything so provocative. She had blonde hair that was curly and fell to just below her shoulders.

The girl exuded raw sexual energy while only sporting a glittery bralette and a black tennis skirt that barely covered her ass cheeks. Additionally, she had an elaborate tattoo of a rose etched on the side of her neck, with thorns extending from the stem and covering the base of her neck in an intricate and complicated pattern.

The blonde started to grin as I watched the females break up their kiss, and I was struck by how much she resembled Natalie Dormer, who portrayed Queen Margaery in Game of Thrones, with her instantly identifiable smirk and light blue eyes that twinkled with mischief and want.

Even in her voice, which was husky and deep like Natalie Dormer's, she said, "Okay, why don't you order the drinks, while I nibble on these for a bit," and as I watched her push the other girl's blazer to the side and start delicately sucking on her nipples, I felt my head start to spin and my heart start to thump in my chest.

We're at a fucking club, Lucy, girl. Pushing Lucy's face away from her breasts, the girl stated, "You can't snack on my nipples like a fucking baby here," before kissing Lucy on the lips to demonstrate that she wasn't being offensive.

Lucy remarked, and the first thing she did was turn back and capture my attention. "Alright, you go ahead and order that drink, while I look around and find the homophobes who have been eyeing us like we are horse shit lying in the middle of the road," she continued.

She caught me off guard, and I knew it because I was looking at her.

I turned my head away and began toying with my hair while clearing my throat for an odd reason in an effort to look casual.

Are you a homophobe like the ones I was mentioning?

I appeared to be unaware of her.

I could no longer hide my awareness of Lucy since she had moved closer to me and was now standing directly in front of me.

I apologized while claiming ignorance, "Sorry?"

The sneer became much more apparent when Lucy grinned.

I suddenly became tense, and I worried whether Lucy could hear the sound of my heart pounding against the wall of my chest over the loud speakers.

In response to her own inquiry, Lucy said, "You are not homophobic; you are just curious, aren't you?"

I'm sorry, but I'm not sure what you mean.

Oh stop the nonsense. I wouldn't have cared if you were homophobic if I could have fucked you. You are one hot lady. From where are you?

I replied, "I am sorry, but I am not a lesbian," since it was the first thing that entered my mind.

Once again laughing, Lucy moved closer to me, nearly touching bodies as she moved her fingers through her hair in the most sensual manner conceivable. Despite the loud music in the club, Lucy murmured, "I would still fuck you, and I would keep fucking you until I turned you into a lesbian, and then you would never go back to sucking dick," leaving me utterly stunned.

"I...I..."

But despite the fact that I would leave her in a heartbeat for a physique like yours, I came here tonight with someone else, and I have a principle. Since I never leave a bar without the person I entered there with, my love, you have just avoided being homosexual. Congratulations. Thankfully, the girl she had come with tapped her shoulder and brought her a drink before Lucy said, "Now you can go back to fucking men and being unsatisfied for the rest of your life." Lucy gazed directly at me, her eyes staying on my face for a few seconds that felt like days to me.

Lucy gave me one final glance that was tinged with curiosity and need before leaving the bar with her hand around the brunette's waist.

I struggled for breath and had to cling onto the bar counter to keep from passing out.

I experienced a quick uprooting, like a powerful wind abruptly uprooting a tree. I was frightened and in total chaos. No one had ever made me feel so anxious and out of breath after only a few seconds of discussion, even though I had been approached by many men and a few women over the years.

I took hold of the whiskey glass that the bartender had just set down for me on the counter and drank the whole thing in one sitting.

My vision of the club was a bit fuzzy, but I knew the alcohol couldn't have begun to affect me so early.

There was another cause for this wooziness. anything I had never previously gone through.

Lesbians, you say? It took me a few seconds to realize what the guy who had been flirting with the lady out of his league had meant when he remarked, "You can't live with 'em, can't live without 'em.

"Pardon me?"

"I overheard that discussion. I don't agree with what the girl stated, and she was highly disrespectful to guys. The guy said, "I believe a man can please a lady like no other woman can. His suit was wrinkled, and the sole hair that was left on his head was uncombed.

I just had to take one look at the guy to realize that Lucy had a far greater chance of meeting my needs than this Lord of the Rings orc.

I told him that I wasn't interested in talking and nodded at the bartender to get me another whiskey glass.

The guy grinned, which made him seem even more repulsive, and said, "You will be if you give me a try.

The boldness of guys to approach women with sleazy pick-up lines, missing teeth, and haircuts that would scream "middle-aged men with superiority complex" was something I could never comprehend.

"Listen, I don't want to speak to you. With me, you are wasting your time.

"I'd be thrilled to squander my time with a lady like you. What if we squander some time in my Rolls Royce, then maybe some more in my Waldorf Astoria room, and finally, after we have spent enough time to get to morning, I can reward you by purchasing you whatever you choose from Tiffany's?

I struggled to control my laughter.

In one minute, the guy had mentioned more products than a Super Bowl ad.

I tried to be a bit more clear this time and answered, "Sorry, not interested," assuming that would be the end of the chat. However, what the guy did next was not at all what I had anticipated.

My wrist was painfully and uncomfortably held in his hold as he twisted me around to face him.

"Listen, I'll give you whatever amount of money you want. more wealth than you've ever experienced. You get what I'm saying, right? The man's voice abruptly changed to one that was menacing and dismal, saying, "Get off your fucking high horse and come with me before you regret passing on the finest fuck of your life.

My body ached from the agony, and I struggled to get out from under his grip, but I was unable to do so because of how tightly he had me held.

Hey, how about I show you the fuck of your life?" Then, for me to understand what was happening, I heard a female voice say.

As the guy let go of my hand and tumbled to the ground, I saw fists fly and one hit just beneath his chin.

I saw Lucy repeatedly kick the guy in the head, leaving blood on the floor while the victim screamed for aid.

Even after being restrained, Lucy struck out at a couple people before they were able to calm her down.

The argument had generated enough disturbance that the DJ had to stop playing the music, and everyone had to stop dancing and crane their necks to observe what had just occurred.

When Lucy glanced at me, all of her wrath vanished and she smiled. When I first saw Lucy, she had untidy blonde hair, boiling anger in her eyes, her chest was beating quickly, and her hands were balled into fists.

She clenched her hands before adjusting her outfit.

Everyone is free to resume dancing now. Other than my badassery, nothing occurred here. If anybody has footage of this on their phone, please give it to me so I can watch it later while having sex.

The girl appeared unmoved by what had transpired, even after getting into a battle and defeating a guy twice her height. Her confidence and lack of emotion were so astounding that I could not help but be in awe of her.

"Are you alright?" Lucy approached me and examined my wrist with both of her hands.

The man's crimson handprint was apparent on the white background of my flesh on my wrists.

I said, "I am okay," and it was only then that I noticed how trembling my voice was.

While touching my wrist and staring into my eyes, Lucy said, "You don't sound okay."

"Who am I kidding, yeah. I said, "I need a drink," as I watched the security carry the guy out of the club.

What the heck did you do to that guy, Lucy? A worried look on her face, the brunette who had been having sex with Lucy emerged from the gathering.

There was "nothing more than what he deserved," Lucy remarked.

"Well, he's kind of a big thing. He is threatening to sue you and owns a chain of hotels on the Upper East Side.

Wonderful, I'm looking forward to it.

"Lucy, you don't get it. He is a very strong guy, and he will certain that he exacts his retribution.

Lucy spun around and looked at the brunette. So Veronica, what do you want me to do? really provide him with the finest fuck of his life?"

118

I want you to apologize to him, not me.

When Lucy laughed, she flung her head back and let out a booming chuckle.

"Check out this cool. Do you think she's real? Lucy questioned me, while pointing to Veronica, Listen up, young lady. If you truly want me to apologize to him, then you can fuck off with him, you get it? No one tells me what to do, okay?

"What? How dare you address me in such a manner? Véronique was furious.

Just leave, listen. Simply leave, Veronica. To be very honest, you are boring as fuck and I am not in the mood for this right now. In any case, I would have abandoned you.

Veronica exhaled, but before she could say anything, she recalled what Lucy had done to the guy and chose not to speak.

Lucy turned to face me and said, "Fuck, guess I'll be sleeping alone tonight."

Despite my want to speak, I was unable to do so since the girl's aura and stunning confidence were so overwhelming.

Lucy questioned, "Are you going to just stand there or are you going to order some drinks for us?"

"I wanted to go out. Clubs are probably not my thing. I remarked, suddenly realizing that I was on the verge of tears.

It took me a while to realize how serious what had just transpired was, and when it did, it left me absolutely without any incentive to change my life as I had imagined I would tonight.

I knew that no matter how hard I tried, I would always be the unattractive girl whose lover left her for someone more interesting and adventurous. I also knew that I was doomed to cry alone in the darkness of my room.

I turned my head aside to try to conceal my face, but Lucy could see the tears running down my cheeks.

I'm sorry, but I'm not very good with words. Although I can tell that you are in pain, is there anything I can do to help?

After wiping away my tears, I turned to face the fiery blonde who was looking at me with worry in her eyes.

Why not take a stroll outside? I don't know what made me say it, but right now I could use someone's company.

I never asked strangers to go on walks with me, but something about Lucy's presence was so reassuring and was giving me such a sense of security that I did not want to let it go so quickly.

Lucy grinned and added, "Seeing as I won't be getting laid tonight, I think I would prefer a walk outside," developing the Natalie Dormer-like smirk at the corner of her lips.

Although the rain had stopped outside, the winds were still strong and carried the smell of wet. As Lucy did next to me, I fastened the buttons on my coat and gave myself a tight embrace.

It was reassuring to realize that, in some ways, she was typical.

Lucy replied, "So, I don't even know your name," as we started to move away from the club and the tiny group of people who were still attempting to enter the club and toward the crossing.

"Amaya," I said.

After Lucy exclaimed, "That is a beautiful name," both of us were quiet.

I am extremely lousy with words, so if we are going on a stroll together, you would have to take the lead in conversation, Lucy stated regretfully. "See, let me tell you something right off the bat, in fact, let me repeat what I have already said," she said.

I grinned and nodded in agreement. "That is okay with me. I questioned, "Where did you learn to fight like that?

I had a difficult upbringing, Lucy stated.

She paused there instead of continuing, which surprised me.

"All right, I suppose you're correct. You don't have that much verbal skill.

No, I don't believe we are close enough for me to elaborate on my upbringing. I'm sorry.

None were taken.

Once there, we came to a halt at a pedestrian-only red signal. A bunch of females arrived and chatted happily while standing next to us.

I murmured, staring wistfully at the females, "I miss this.

"What?"

"Just relaxing with friends and not giving a damn about anything."

Don't get me wrong, but what's keeping you from doing it right now?

I grinned mischievously and added, "I don't think we are close enough for me to tell you that, Miss Wonder Woman," as the light went green and we crossed the street.

The wind was screaming all around us, and our jackets were fluttering around our ankles. For the first time in months, I felt a slight tingle between my legs, which I was able to hide, but it was enough to send my mind into overdrive. The traffic was light, the night sky was dotted with twinkling points of silver light, shining overhead with all their beauty. Then, my eyes fell upon Lucy's face and her stunning blue eyes.

Why was this happening?

"Okay. The flavor of my own medication did not appeal to me. However, based on the little time I've had with you, I've come to the conclusion that you're not the sort of lady who does this often. You come out as a sweet lady who enjoys watching the Bachelorette at home while daydreaming about being hitched to a dashing guy.

I laughed out loud.

A genuine chuckle that comes from the heart had long since been absent from my existence.

I was a girl like that. I suppose I still am, but I had hoped to rectify that today before everything went awry.

When she turned to face me and said, "The night is still young, Amaya," Lucy continued, "If you want, I can still show you the night of your life."

I said, "I'm straight, Lucy."

Oh, I understand, and even though I would have liked it if you weren't, I am not just interested in sex.

"Yes, I am aware. You also like gory beatings of males.

Yes, it is true, but I also value having fun. I may be able to salvage this night for you if you give me the opportunity.

I grabbed Lucy by the waist and yanked her to the side, warning her to be careful since there was a pole behind her.

However, I dragged her harder than I meant to, crashing our bodies against one another.

Lucy fell into my arms and supported herself by grabbing my waist.

While Lucy smiled at me and made no attempt to let go of me, I kept her in that position for a short period of time.

In the end, I had to let her go, and Lucy laughed like a little girl as I did.

You once rescued me, and now I've saved you. We are equal.

As we approached another crossing, with a sizable electronic billboard lighting up the square and covering the road in a tapestry of vibrant colors, Lucy joked, "Yes, I am sure that pole would have put up a very good fight if only it wasn't a non-living object. So what do you say, Amaya? Are you willing to assist me in rescuing you this evening?

I came to a complete stop and turned to gaze up at one of the billboards that was promoting the release of the most recent Taylor Swift single.

What comes to mind when I ask? I enquired as the word "Lover" from her next song appeared across the screen.

Lucy grinned and added, "I won't tell you, but I can show you, and for that, we will have to go back to the club."

***

I shook my head and took a step back from the BMW S 1000RR, a superbike that was louder than any other bike I had ever heard. "No fucking way," I exclaimed.

Lucy, who was sat on the bike, straddling the seat like a professional racer, leaning forward over the gasoline tank, and seeming to be the most sexist thing on the earth, urged Amaya to get on. "Amaya, believe me, just hop on, and I promise you will not regret it," she said.

It made me wonder if there was anything this girl couldn't accomplish as I stepped back and gazed at her, admiring her legs, her small waist, and her blonde hair playing with the wind as she sat on the superbike.

I guarantee that nothing will happen to you if you closely hold on to me, Lucy added.

As opposed to choosing death and not holding you?"

Saying, "Amaya, just hop on, babe."

I didn't like riding bikes, especially ones that weren't designed to travel at speeds lower than a hundred miles per hour, but when I imagined sitting behind Lucy, grabbing her by the waist, and pressing up against her body as she led me off to who knows where, my heart began to race with nervous excitement.

"All right, all right, I'll do this, but only if you promise to slow down when I ask you to," the driver said.

"Amaya, whenever girls ask me to slow down, it only makes me want to go faster...and harder."

I grinned wryly.

Why must everything be made sexual, I ask you? I questioned while uncomfortably throwing myself onto the backset.

"With that height, I think you would look so hot riding this bike," Lucy added as she put on her helmet and handed one to me.

I said, "I don't think my dress was made to be worn on bikes," since my whole left leg was exposed by the thigh-high slit of my skirt.

My legs caught Lucy's attention as she moved her head to look at them.

A few moments passed into a minute, and Lucy did nothing except continue to ogle my legs.

"Pardon me? When can we leave? I questioned, a little hesitant.

I'm sorry, but your legs are the sexiest I've ever seen. Are you certain that you aren't even somewhat gay?

I responded, "Just go, Lucy," trying to cover off my flushing cheeks.

"All right, take hold of my waist and keep it tight. This will be a good journey, I can tell."

The cop questioned Stella, "When did the man first knock on your door?"

It was probably about one in the morning.

The knocking "Was it aggressive?"

"Yes, there was no knocking at all. It resembled thumping more. Even though I was already sleeping, I got out of bed nonetheless because I was too afraid and sweaty to even try to open the door. Stella said, still clearly startled, "I was afraid my door might fall off the hinges.

Okay, are you sure that was your old employer? said the police officer taking notes.

"Yes."

The question is, "How do you know that?"

"Because I am familiar with both his voice and appearance. Stella brushed her hair back and looked about the room cautiously as if the intruder was still hiding there. "I saw him through the peephole," she said.

What happened after you requested that he leave?

He promised not to till I unlocked the door. He promised to knock on the door before entering and having his way with me.

The second officer gave a shrug, put his shoulder to his partner's, and spoke softly into his ear.

"Why did you leave your position at the restaurant?"

"Had I not told you before? I used to flirt with the restaurant's owner, Mark, but one day he became physical and attempted to kiss me. I pleaded with him to stop, but he refused. I was only kept alive when a client arrived. The following day, I gave up. He's been phoning my phone ever since, threatening to rape me and to break into my flat if I didn't comply with his demands.

The question that he posed was, "And what was he asking?"

"To have a sexual relationship with me."

The two policemen exchanged glances before the one in front of Stella inhaled deeply and said, "Ma'am, we understand that the night has been very traumatic for you, but you also need to understand that we cannot arrest this man without any evidence. We currently just have your word, and the individual in issue has considerable power in the city.

Stella let out a frustrated groan.

"But I told you, he used to call me from unknown numbers, and I forgot to record the conversation. And tonight, when he came to my door, there was no way I could record him without opening the door and putting myself in danger. And I'm poor, so I don't live in a building with CCTV cameras."

The policeman said, "We understand, but we really can't go and arrest him on your word.

"So, what's the plan of action? Simply remain here till he returns and rapes me?

The officers exchanged puzzled looks with one another before handing Stella a piece of paper with a number written on it.

Stella questioned, "What is this?"

"This is Officer Peyton's personal line. She is a member of the neighborhood precinct and only lives two streets away. Call this number if you feel threatened; she will arrive more quickly than any of us can and is an expert in situations much like yours.

Stella examined the piece of paper in her palm, feeling little let down by the police department's reaction.

"Will you take appropriate action then if I have proof that this man is harassing me?"

Yes, provided the proof is convincing enough.

Stella spoke to the police officer who was looking straight at her cleavage and remarked, "I can't say I am pleased, officers.

The policeman stood up from Stella's crimson sofa. "We are sorry you feel that way, but if we were to go around arresting every man just on the word of a woman who is as hot as you, then we would be out of space in our jails," he remarked.

What does it imply, exactly? Stella was indignant.

"You are aware of its full meaning. In the future, don't squander our time. Stella was left in a state of shock and rage as the two officers left the residence after saying "have a good day."

***

Stella had trouble falling asleep since the wind was roaring outside, and her neighbors were up at 4 in the morning watching an old Clint Eastwood film.

Every time the wind raged outside and sent a loose metal scrap or beer cans flying through the streets below, Stella would toss and turn with visions of Mark, tormenting her with flashes of his face, with rage and lust in his eyes, and revenge on his mind.

Stella clenched the piece of paper with the officer's number closer to her heart as her anxiety and terror increased.

She eventually reached her breaking point and slouched down on the sofa with the paper still in her hand after

135

getting up and entering her living room/kitchen.

Do I need to contact her? What if it's unsuitable? Yet isn't it part of her job? Isn't she more likely to comprehend my predicament since she is a woman?

Stella's mind began to race, and she debated whether or not to phone this Officer Peyton.

Finally, her hands dialed the number on her mobile phone as her fear took over.

Stella's phone rang for a while until a very seductive, velvety female voice answered it just as she was about to lose hope of hearing back.

"Hello?"

Is this Officer Peyton on the line? "Hello, hello, uh.

The voice on the other end questioned, "Yes you are, how can I help you?"

Stella questioned how the lady could be so kind at four in the morning.

"I'm not sure how to say this, but a police officer who works with you gave me your number. Tonight, I had a break-in, and after the burglar departed after a failed effort, I phoned the police. However, the policemen were very useless and impolite. They did, however, offer me your phone number and instructed me to contact you if I had any issues, and I'm afraid, Officer. Both the weather outside and the guy who is pursuing me are quite ominous. He is threatening to rape me, and I have a sense he will keep acting this way because he knows people in the police department. I was expecting that because you are a woman, you would understand my plight and kindly assist me.

Stella could hear nothing on the other end, and her chest tightened as a result.

The question "Where do you live?"

Stella replied, "23, Avelon Street," unsure of what the lady would do with this information.

"Can I come see you right away?"

Indeed, but you're not required to. The hour is really late, and...

"Don't stress about it. I have left. You take precautions and are unconcerned about anything. The fact that you phoned me was a wonderful thing. The lady assured her that everything would be okay before disconnecting the call. Stella later recognized that the officer had done more to reassure her over the phone than the other cops had in more than an hour.

Stella heard a knock on her front door, and for a brief moment, she was terrified. However, she soon recognized that the tap was subtle and not at all threatening.

Stella approached the front door and peered through the peephole to see a young girl with black hair pulled back into a ponytail and very attractive features waiting for a response.

Stella inquired without flinging open the door, "Who is it?"

"This is Police Officer Peyton."

When Stella learned it, she was a little taken aback.

How could an officer be as handsome and young?

Stella felt her heart skip a beat as she opened the door and beheld the young

Officer for the first time in all her magnificence.

Hello, I believe you are the one who called, Peyton enquired.

Stella motioned for Peyton to enter her one-bedroom apartment while stepping to the side. "Yes, please come in, Officer," she replied.

Stella watched as this young, stunning girl who had just entered her home grinned, said a "thank you," and entered.

The girl's height caught Stella's attention right away.

Stella estimated Peyton to be at least 5 feet and 10 inches tall, and when she turned around to face her once inside, Stella's eyes fell on her face, which was both attractive and youthful, with big brown eyes, thick, arched eyebrows, a small, pointed nose, full, juicy lips, and black hair pulled back in a high ponytail. The girl resembled a supermodel more than a police officer.

The girl's figure was out of this world when she wore low-cut white tank top and denim trousers.

Her cleavage protruded from her tank top due to her large breasts, toned arms, petite yet well shaped hips, and hefty breasts.

For a few wonderful minutes, Stella simply stood and gazed at this beauty, forgetting her worries and fears, until Peyton broke her spell by inquiring as to where they should sit.

Stella smiled and replied, "I believe you would be comfortable on the sofa.

Stella followed Peyton, nodding as she moved towards the sofa before pausing to examine herself in the wall mirror next to the front entrance.

Stella was aware of her attractiveness and, at the age of 36, felt she had done well to keep her appearance. She had light golden hair, blue eyes, and the curves of a dancer.

She was often referred to as "Shakira" by her pals because of her curly hair and superior belly dancing abilities.

Stella apologized profusely for bothering her at this time.

"That's okay, I was just getting off work. In any case, I would have chosen a 9 to 5 job if I sought comfort at work.

Stella tried her best not to swoon over Peyton's cleavage as she continued, "If only the policemen that showed up at my door carried the same attitude like you."

"I apologize for their actions. I don't know what they did, but I'm sure they must have been a major pain in the ass," Peyton replied, and despite the girl's youth, there was an air of authority and self-assurance in her voice that intimidated.

"Yes, they were," Stella acknowledged.

Say, "So tell me, what happened?"

Stella started off by recounting the whole scenario, starting with how the owner had once visited the franchise where she had worked at Marco's, one of the largest Italian restaurant chains in the state, and how she had been employed as a server there.

After many days of stalking and harassment, there was ultimately an attempt at rape as a result of that.

When Stella eventually described the incident with the officers, Peyton's face began to become redder and her nostrils began to flare. Despite the fact that Stella knew the girl was becoming agitated, she was unable to help but note how much more attractive the girl seemed with her cheeks red.

Peyton crossed her knees and shook her head, "This is just crap.

Stella was puzzled as to how to react, but she was relieved that someone had seen her and understood her annoyance.

Listen, I'll have my Sergeant give me your case, and I'll make sure you're secure. Stella's heart went into overdrive when Peyton added, "Don't you worry about that," while maintaining her hand briefly on her thigh.

Why is this girl making me feel this way?

I simply want to stay secure, therefore I'm just happy that someone from the authorities took me seriously.

"You will be. I live barely five minutes away, and I will be here before you know it. I do understand this man is a big deal, and even I won't be able to function like I normally do."

Yes, I am aware of it.

Things were a bit odd when Stella became quiet.

Stella up from the sofa and offered to make the man a cup of coffee.

"That won't be necessary, Ma'am. I have to go back and go to sleep, plus if I drink coffee, then I would be up the whole day," the person said.

You have been so helpful, I can't simply let you leave without a drink. Well, I can certainly need one, and I would appreciate it if you could offer me some company.

Peyton hurried over and said, "Do you have whiskey?"

I really do, in fact. Stella made her way from the living area to her open kitchen. "I don't typically drink whiskey myself, but I had a friend over who is a big whiskey fan," she remarked.

"Are you a single person?", Peyton inquired as Stella searched her wine cupboard.

"Yeah, I used to have a roommate, but she was kind of a maniac, so I had to get rid of her. While I was looking for a new one, I discovered I preferred living alone.

Peyton said, "I live alone as well," and Stella could just make out a hint of melancholy in her tone.

"Officer, what's your age?"

Stella found Peyton's laughter to be utter joy to her ears.

"I often hear this from folks. I am 24. Yes, I am a bit young, but I excelled in my class at the Police Academy and was given a promotion before others.

As Stella located the Jack Daniels bottle, she grinned.

"I understand why. I can already see you have a bright future from the way you are treating my case.

Stella arrived with two glasses and the whiskey bottle, set them on the wooden center table, and then sat down.

Peyton said, "I assumed you were preparing a cup of coffee for yourself.

Stella responded, "I think I need alcohol more than I need caffeine," and shrugged.

If you weren't in such a weak position, I would be hitting on you right now. What a freaking gorgeous lady you are!' Peyton pondered as she observed Stella's curves and the fact that every time she smiled, two little dimples emerged on her face. Peyton was also a bit of a nymphomaniac since she could already feel moisture on the front of her underwear.

If you're so young, why do you live alone? Stella poured a drink for them both and added, "I thought females your age preferred living together, partying all the time, getting intoxicated, and making out with each other.

When females were mentioned having sex, Peyton's ears pricked up and she felt she would really have a shot.

Yes, I do all of those things, but I prefer that my ladies go the next morning.

Stella was about to take a drink when she abruptly halted, the glass coming dangerously close to her lips.

"Girls?"

Yes, I'm homosexual. I like ladies.

Stella's eyes briefly darted from Peyton's face to various locations around her apartment, and she briefly experienced stomach butterflies.

Oh, then, it only makes having a roommate even more logical. That isn't the ultimate dream, is it?"

"I can't tell you how many times I've done it. Right now, I simply need something steady. I've been using Tinder, and although it may be entertaining at first, you soon realize that after the excitement wears off, you are left alone and have no one with whom to share your joy, your suffering, or your triumphs. Sorry, I'm rambling now.

"No, no problem. I assume you have pals.

But they are all just like me, yeah. They are occupied leading emotionless lives.

Stella replied, "I mean, you're a policewoman and I can see you truly care about people, especially women, but you seem so cautious when it comes to a long-term commitment with someone.

"Yup, I guess I'm a bit odd. Ma'am, how about you? If I'm not mistaken, you must be in your late twenties."

You are mistaken, Stella remarked while grinning and gulping down her whiskey. I am 36."

"What? You don't seem to be it! You are so lovely. I briefly believed I had entered Shakira's residence.

"Yes, because Shakira wouldn't be living in a one-bedroom apartment without CCTVs."

Peyton chuckled as she drank her whiskey.

"Ma'am, you seem like an intriguing person. Peyton added, "I would want to get to know you better. I understand how direct and abrupt that sounded, and I inwardly scolded myself.

"I humbly disagree. You intrigue me far more, in my opinion. a young woman in her early 20s who works as a police officer, lives alone, and engages in one-night encounters with females. There isn't a single person I know that is even remotely close to being as fascinating as you.

"Okay, that's excellent. Let's get together again, maybe under better conditions, as we live near by. Hopefully the dude won't disturb you again.

As Peyton stated this, Stella's memory of what had happened earlier in the evening returned. She realized that this attractive, young cop would soon go, leaving her once again alone and a potential target for one of the city's most powerful men.

Yes, I do hope so as well.

"All right, Ma'am, you may now go. You have my phone number, so please don't be hesitant to contact me at any moment. I am always available to you.

First off, please stop addressing me as Ma'am. We had just recently become pals, I thought.

Okay, Stella," Peyton remarked with emphasis on Stella's name.

Be careful, Peyton.

Yes, Shakira, you too!"

***

a day later. Stella made the decision to stay in bed all day. She was not in a rush to obtain a work and yet did not have a job to go to. She had too much going on in her life to add the burden of another job on top of it all.

However, the most recent development that had intrigued her was her body's reaction to Peyton, the attractive young policewoman who had been such a sweetheart to her the previous evening.

She couldn't help but go back to how her heart had skipped a beat when she had first seen the girl, and how the girl had captured her ever since as she lay in bed, bundled in covers, with her laptop on her belly, and "Friends" running on the screen.

Stella was intrigued by everything about her—from the way she sat to the way she moved, her eyes, her high ponytail, her self-assurance and personality, her life narrative, and the fact that she was attracted to women.

Do I also have an interest in women? However, this has never occurred before. Why this girl then?

When Stella had kissed a girl in college at a frat party, she recalled that she had felt absolutely nothing. The sex had always been amazing, even while she was married to her ex-husband, and she had never felt the need to approach females for her sexual demands.

Yes, she sometimes enjoyed the feminine beauty, but more as an admirer than as someone who desired to have a sexual relationship with them.

But now that ideas had started to permeate her mind, she finally considered what it may be like to have her first lesbian encounter with this attractive, dominant policewoman who was used to sleeping with a new woman every day.

She suddenly became aware that she was moist once again.

***

Stella arrived home with the idea of climbing into her bed and falling asleep for a while after going for a stroll down to her neighborhood grocery shop to pick up a few things.

Thankfully, neither Mark nor any of his guys had made an effort to get in touch with her despite the fact that she had a lot on her mind all day.

He may have concluded it was not worth it because he was over her, because he knew the police were now involved, or because he was just waiting for the appropriate opportunity.

After a small pasta meal, Stella had a lengthy bath. At times, she felt the want to touch her pussy as she thought about Peyton, but she restrained herself.

She was not going to behave like that. The girl was very youthful for her age—she was 36.

Although it would be inappropriate for her to consider her sexually, she intuitively knew it would also make her feel wonderful.

Stella was prepared to go asleep after fighting dirty thoughts about Peyton in the shower.

She attempted to fall asleep with the window open so she could see the night sky and the full moon.

She didn't take long to go into the realm of dreams, where she also ran across Peyton.

She could plainly see the young officer laying next to her in bed, facing her with her legs draped over her torso and her eyes boring a hole through her soul while her pussy throbbed with want.

Stella saw the protection of the girls' arms as a vibranium shield in her dreams as she watched the two of them holding firmly and pressing their bodies together.

Stella cried out in her sleep at some point throughout the course of the night, experiencing the effects of Peyton kissing her lips in her fantasies but not in reality.

Stella was sleeping more deeper than she anticipated and was so engrossed in her sleep that she was oblivious to the sound of a guy climbing through her window and lightly landing on the floor of her bedroom.

The guy leaned over the sleeping blonde while donning a mask and a black sweatshirt. His lips twisted into a grin.

Stella grinned as he ran his finger over the woman's hair, thinking it was Peyton.

The guy stood over the lady and waited as a blast of wind entered through the window and the curtains danced merrily.

He couldn't decide.

Should he grab her and tie her up right away, or should he wait for her to get up so he can savour the look of panic on her face before he has his way with her?

Stella moved slightly in her sleep and slightly opened her eyes, but what she saw caused her to startle up and sit on her bed with wide eyes.

The man's voice was muffled as he spoke, "Hello, Stella," making it obvious that he had gone to considerable measures to keep his identity a secret from Stella.

Stella, though, was already starting to perspire.

She had no clue what to do since her biggest dread had manifested sooner than she had anticipated.

Who are you?"Stella questioned in a trembling voice.

"I am the stuff of nightmares. You ought to have given Boss free rein. He would have promoted you and maybe purchased you a new vehicle, purse, or pair of shoes. But since you had to be a bit cautious, look where it's gotten us today."

Stella was aware that Mark was not the guy who was now in her bedroom.

Mark wasn't this big or as muscular as he seemed.

Stella was aware that even if Peyton were to barge into the room at this very moment, the guy in it would have the physique of a powerlifter.

Whoever you are, pay attention. This won't get away from you. Police are aware. If something were to happen to me, they would inquire about your boss since I have given them the whole tale.

"Let them interrogate him. He'll claim that nothing of the kind ever took place, and I'll be gone on an island with the cash he'll give me for fucking your brains out. Yes, I'll fuck you, I assure you. I will take pleasure in it. Since I first saw you dressed as a waitress, I have had my eyes on you. Damn, their hips had me in such a bind. That night, I blew a large nut in your face, and now, you slut, I'm going to blow a nut within you.

Stella bolted from the room as the guy put his knee on the edge of the bed.

She sprang from the bed and ran for the door, but the guy caught up to her in two steps, grabbed her by the back, and then threw her on the bed.

Stella was anticipating the worst as her heart was racing.

She wanted to scream and tears were already flowing down her cheeks, but she was being suffocated by something.

She was having trouble breathing and was on the verge of passing out.

After giving up on attempting to escape, Stella simply gave up as the guy got into the bed, grabbed her by the hair, and pulled her head back.

Stella groaned in agony, her body limping and her eyes becoming black.

Possibly now.

If it occurred while she was unconscious, that would be preferable.

His lips were on hers, and she felt her hands fumbling through her nightgown for her breasts.

Then it took place.

Her thoughts started to race, and eventually the blackness swallowed her.

But just as she started to lose awareness of her surroundings, she heard a loud, clear sound.

A gunshot had just been fired.
***

She could hear a deep, beautiful voice in her ear. A voice from last night that had become her ally.

When Stella opened her eyes, she saw her room's ceiling.

When she tilted her head to the side, Peyton was seated on the bed next to her, wearing an off-the-shoulder shirt and a short black checkered skirt.

Hey, you dare not stand up. Go on lying.

"Peyton?Stella was able to say, ".

Yes, I am present. The situation is good. Nothing should bother you. You should get more rest.

"Th..The...M..Man?"

"I looked after him. Peyton pointed a pistol at him and screamed, "Shoot him with this.

You murdered him?"

"I wish I could, but I couldn't. He was wounded in the kneecap.

Stella's eyesight was still hazy, but even in a state of shock and mental tiredness, she could make out how hot Peyton looked in her skirt and top,

157

clutching the pistol like a badass but yet appearing extremely feminine.

I need to sleep, Stella said, closing her eyes once again and falling asleep.

***

Stella felt a strong flash of melancholy when she opened her eyes this time and realized Peyton was not there to greet her. The girl had she left? So soon after everything she had gone through, was she alone.

Stella decided it was time to make an effort to get up, and after feeling lightheaded for a while, she left her room and found Peyton on the red sofa reading a book and holding a drink of whiskey.

Stella joined Peyton on the sofa, but this time sat beside her rather than in front of her. "I am glad you are still here," she remarked.

She was immediately entranced by Peyton's presence once again as soon as she smelt her perfume and saw her lovely brown eyes as he sat down.

Why did I have to leave you? Remember, we're pals.How are you feeling right now?" Peyton grinned."

I'm glad you're here, if a bit dizzy and unsettled.

"You've told me that twice now," I said.

I am so glad to see you, it's beyond words. And I'm not sure how to express my gratitude for what you accomplished. How, specifically, did you know that he would appear the next day?"

"I asked my friend to watch out for him. He observed him leave one of his locations and drive right into your area, but instead of getting out, a large, black guy exited and began up the fire escape. I suppose Mark had hired him to essentially do whatever he wanted. My partner contacted me at that point, and I arrived as quickly as I could. Mark was nowhere to be found. He probably departed once he learned what had transpired.

"What ever become of the guy you shot?"

"I phoned again and had him taken into custody. He is now in prison, and I shall question him shortly. I would have completed it today, but I just didn't want to leave you.

When Stella heard it, her heart warmed. Even though she was now certain that she had a serious crush on this young girl, she was unsure of how to handle it.

"Peyton, you are a wonderful guy. Stella sobbed, "You literally saved my life," before abruptly letting her feelings overwhelm her and hugging Peyton.

Surprised by Stella's unexpected display of emotion, Peyton embraced her back. Feeling her pussy twitch, Peyton smelt Stella's hair and suppressed the want to simply grab Stella and give her a passionate kiss.

Stella let Peyton move at her own leisurely pace. She struggled mightily to let go of Peyton once she had her in her arms, and never before had she embraced a girl while feeling so compelled to kiss her.

The young officer finally grinned widely as Stella let Peyton go, which was something she did not often. She then flushed, which was once again a highly unusual event for the young, self-assured, and generally serious girl.

Stella said, "I see that you did manage to find your way to my liquor cabinet."

Yes, I required it. Peyton sipped on her drink while staring intently at Stella. "I always get a little too excited and horny after shooting someone," she stated.

Oh my gosh, it is both terrifying and seductive. I can't be anything else right now because I'm too anxious. My body may just have forgotten how to feel aroused because I haven't had sex in a year.

Peyton surprisedly opened her lips, kept the beverage on the table, and leaned back on the couch.

You haven't had sexual contact in a year?"

"Yeah, never found any god enough or attractive guys."

"Are you certain that you have no interest in women as well?"

Stella said, "I think I might just be," realizing that her boldness was out of character.

"Oh. Is there a method to determine that?"

"I'm not sure,"

We can visit a lesbian pub to check if you have a crush on somebody."

Stella chuckled and shook her head, saying, "There is no way I am doing that."

Why not?""

"Since...I'm not sure. I believe the only way I'll know for sure is to test it out on a friend. someone I really like or feel at ease with."

"Drinking alcohol may quickly make you feel at ease with anybody. Look, I've made up my mind to take you to a bar. I may not be at a lesbian club, but I feel like I could need some fresh air.

Stella hesitated because she was still quite afraid of Mark hiding outside, in a trash, or around a corner.

What is the issue?"

"I'm scared,"

But I'll be there with you. Stella was astounded by how hot and fierce this lady looked while shouting and carrying a pistol in her hand. "And I am taking this with you, and believe me, the next time, I won't aim for the motherfucker's knees," Peyton added.

She experienced a level of arousal beyond what she had anticipated.

Stella just answered, "Alright, let's go," since she wanted to spend as much time with Peyton as she could.